I0824562

Praise for *The Truth About Seed Oils*

"We've been lied to for far too long about what's in our food, and this book helps expose the truth about one of the biggest deceptions of all: seed oils. This book is a powerful wake-up call, reminding us that real food and unadulterated fat are the foundation of health. When people are given the truth, they're empowered to make better choices, and education like this is how real change begins."

—**Vani Hari**, *New York Times* bestselling author of *The Food Babe Kitchen* and founder of Truvani

"There's a lot of confusion today about fats and seed oils, and this book brings much needed clarity to an often-misunderstood topic. I've seen firsthand how choosing the right fats can dramatically impact inflammation, energy levels, gut health, and overall wellness, and this book empowers people to make those changes with confidence."

—**Dr. Josh Axe**, *New York Times* bestselling author and founder of Ancient Nutrition

"In my telehealth practice, I've seen people's health dramatically improve when they remove industrial seed oils —from clearer skin and stronger hair to better gut health and reduced chronic inflammation and arthritis pain. *The Truth About Seed Oils* explains why this happens and empowers readers with practical, nourishing recipes to create real, lasting change."

—**Dr. Will Cole**, leading functional medicine expert and *New York Times* bestselling author

"This book boldly challenges decades of misinformation that have made us sick and tired and replaces it with truth rooted in biology and ancestral wisdom. *The Truth About Seed Oils* empowers readers to understand what's really harming their bodies—and how simple dietary shifts can restore energy, metabolic health, and hope. A must-read for anyone serious about real wellness."

—**Dr. Austin Lake**

"For decades, we've been told a simple story: vegetable oils are 'heart-healthy,' saturated fat is dangerous, and the science is settled. But when you actually look at people's health—rising inflammation, insulin resistance, chronic fatigue, and metabolic disease—it's clear something doesn't add up. What I appreciate about this book is its clarity. Cherie Calbom and Liana Werner-Gray cut through the confusion and get straight to the root cause. They explain why these oils are problematic, how they damage the body, and—most importantly—what to do instead. This isn't about fear; it's about replacing unstable, inflammatory fats with real, traditional fats the body actually recognizes and knows how to use. If you're serious about healing inflammation, restoring energy, and taking control of your health, this is an important place to start."

—**Dr. Eric Berg, DC**, leading health educator and bestselling author of *The Healthy Keto Plan* and *The 7 Principles of Fat Burning*

"We are called to be good stewards of the bodies God has entrusted to us, yet so many well-meaning people are confused and misled when it comes to nutrition. Seed oils may be one of the most misunderstood trends of our time, and this book brings much-needed truth and clarity. Written by trusted, bestselling authors who have spent years researching this topic, it gently but boldly helps separate fact from fiction while offering real hope. What I appreciate most is that this book doesn't just explain what's wrong—it goes a step further and shows us how to move forward with practical guidance and delicious recipes that make healthy change feel doable. This is an encouraging, empowering resource for anyone who wants to honor God, care for their health, and live and heal strong with wisdom and understanding."

—**Suzy Griswold, MPH**, founder of HealingStrong

"*The Truth About Seed Oils* is a powerful, practical guide for anyone ready to heal at the cellular level. This book goes beyond the science and delivers beautiful, nourishing recipes that are blood-sugar balanced, gut-loving, low-toxin, and anti-inflammatory. These are the kinds of meals that look indulgent, yet quietly support your liver, mitochondria, hormones, and nervous system, using mineral rich spices, clean fats, quality protein, and gentle acids that aid digestion rather than stress it. A must-read (and must-cook) for real, sustainable healing."

—**Dr. Jess Peatross**

THE TRUTH ABOUT SEED OILS

HOW THE "HEART-HEALTHY" MYTH MADE US SICK—AND HOW TO HEAL WITH REAL FATS

LIANA WERNER-GRAY

AND

CHERIE CALBOM, MS

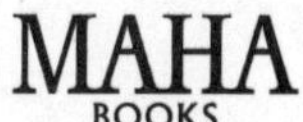

A portion of the proceeds goes to MAHA Action 501(c)4.

MAHA Books may be purchased in bulk at special discounts for sales promotion, corporate gifts, fund-raising, or educational purposes. Special editions can also be created to specifications. For details, contact the Special Sales Department, Skyhorse Publishing, 307 Fifth Avenue, 4th Floor, New York, NY 10016 or info@skyhorsepublishing.com.

MAHA Books is an imprint of Skyhorse Publishing, Inc.®, a Delaware corporation.

Visit our website at www.skyhorsepublishing.com.

Please follow our publisher Tony Lyons on Instagram @tonylyonsisuncertain.

10 9 8 7 6 5 4 3 2 1

Library of Congress Cataloging-in-Publication Data is available on file.

Cover design by David Ter-Avanesyan
Cover image by Getty Images

Print ISBN: 978-1-63144-100-4
Ebook ISBN: 978-1-63144-101-1

Printed in the United States of America

This book is dedicated to those seeking the truth even when it challenges everything they were told.

Disclaimer

The information in this book is intended for educational purposes only and is not a substitute for personalized medical advice. Nutrition is highly bio-individual, and what works well for one person may not work for another.

As nutritionists with decades of clinical experience, we have worked with a wide range of individuals. For some people, traditional fats such as grass-fed butter, beef tallow, or other animal fats can be supportive and nourishing. For others, depending on genetics, digestion, inflammation, hormone balance, or underlying health conditions, those same fats may not be well tolerated and can contribute to digestive or inflammatory reactions. In certain cases, a greater focus on plant-based fats may be more appropriate, while for others, particularly those with specific neurological or metabolic needs, wild-caught fatty fish and grass-fed beef may be beneficial.

It is important to listen to your body, practice discernment, and honor your unique physiology. Food sensitivity testing or working with a qualified healthcare practitioner can provide additional insight. While individual fat tolerance varies, the evidence is clear that highly processed industrial seed oils are not supportive of human health. The goal of this book is to help you make informed, empowered choices and return to real, whole foods that align with your body's needs.

Contents

Introduction:	Rethinking Familiar Oils	ix
Chapter 1:	Liquid Lies: The Seed Oil Scandal	1
Chapter 2:	Seed Oils Cause Anxiety, Depression, Cancer, Alzheimer's, Dementia, and Worse	25
Chapter 3:	Everything You Need to Know About Oils and Fats	46
Chapter 4:	Nourishing Recipes with Nature's Healthiest Fats and Oils	65
Chapter 5:	The Good Fats and Oils Shopping Guide and Resources	129
About the Authors		137
Acknowledgments		138
Endnotes		139
Index		147

INTRODUCTION
Rethinking Familiar Oils

There's a lot of confusion and questions concerning fats and oils. Science says that canola is the best oil to cook with, right? Is coconut oil artery-clogging? Should we use an alternative spread instead of butter? Isn't beef tallow dangerous to use? *The Truth About Seed Oils* brings clarity to a jungle of misinformation. We'll show you how seed oils are silent killers. These oils, also known as the "hateful eight," are responsible for untold numbers of chronic diseases, as we show in chapter 2. Yet we don't see what they are doing as they silently destroy our health. The good news is that a few simple changes can turn that around and set you on a path to good health and disease prevention.

Recently, Liana's friend shared that she was eager to learn more about just how harmful seed oils may be, especially after her grandmother insisted she "needed canola oil to help her heart." Not long after, Cherie and her husband went out to dinner with friends, where the topic of beef tallow unexpectedly came up. Steak 'n Shake had been in the news for switching its frying fat to beef tallow, prompting the question: Why would they do that? Isn't that bad for your heart? A lively discussion followed, with canola oil confidently defended as a healthy cooking choice. What struck us most wasn't just the debate itself, but how deeply these beliefs were held and how widespread the confusion had become. It was clear to us that it was time to set the record straight about seed oils—and we know this book will do just that.

What do you consider to be the components of a healthy lifestyle? Avoiding animal fats? Cooking with vegetable oils because they're "heart-healthy"? Avoiding all saturated fat: no butter, steak, or beef tallow? What if it all were false?

Vegetable oils, now known as seed oils, surround us—in packaged foods, at restaurants, and drizzled onto salads. They are the oils recommended by your doctor and have long been endorsed by the American Heart Association—we will get more into that later. Seed oils are abundant in a typical American diet, including canola (also known as rapeseed oil) and soybean oils, as well as corn, safflower, grapeseed, and sunflower oils. Yet most people know very little about how they are made, why they became popular (hint: follow the money), why they are toxic, and how they harm the body.

These oils appear to be the epitome of health, but that is where we often make a wrong assumption. Chemically refined, deodorized, and heat-treated, they are anything but healthy. This production cycle produces volatile oxidized oils. When they break down into unstable forms, they produce toxic by-products. The high heat used in manufacturing alters the structure of fats, leading to lipid peroxidation, in which fats react with oxygen to form free radicals, reactive aldehydes, and lipid peroxides. Free radicals can damage cells, proteins, and DNA, thus contributing to oxidative stress and inflammation. This is linked to weight gain, including obesity, metabolic dysfunction, chronic inflammation, cancer, depression, diabetes, dementia, heart disease, and numerous other chronic diseases, as you will learn about in the book.

In chapter 1, we will take a look at the dark history of seed oils, which were never created for their health benefits. You will learn why seed oils were created in the first place. You will find out what caused food manufacturers to resort to deceptive practices and promote products and practices that actually harmed the health of this nation. And you'll understand why an ingredient list made up of inflammatory, rancid seed oils was promoted to the public in the first place.

When ethics take a back seat to profit, greed takes the driver's seat. If taste, seduction, and profitability are the imperatives, health concern is lost. Secretary of Health and Human Services Robert F. Kennedy Jr.

said it's a spiritual problem. The spiritual connection to the source of our food is severed in the face of greed. This deception can be seen as a moral flaw—an assault on integrity and honesty. How did we lose our way? This goes back to losing the link to our source of all life. For generations, people believed food, rain, soil, and sunshine were gifts from God. Food was a blessing from our Creator. Part of having a healthy relationship with food was acknowledging and appreciating that gift. People gave thanks for their food before each meal. Our connection with the divine is broken when food is robbed of its natural intentions and is no longer a whole food. The meal of today is not a holy gift, but an economic commodity.

Do you think big businesses in the seed oil market, which is projected to reach $598 billion by 2031, view people as "made in the likeness and image of God?" They want you to continue to be part of helping run their economic engine. The body is not seen as sacred and therefore can be trashed with toxic foods that destroy health. A return to healthy fats and oils can be seen as a return to what God gave us for our good.

The Truth About Seed Oils is the story of edible oils and fats. It's a return to the spiritual aspect of real food. It pulls back the curtain on decades of hype and flawed, incomplete, or even fraudulent research that has taken us down this path. The truth is that seed oils are beyond harmful for us, while we've been ignoring, even demonizing, truly healthy fats and oils, such as beef tallow and coconut oil. Additionally, eliminating seed oils from our diet can be one of the most significant steps we can take for our health. Understanding the truth about fats and oils isn't rocket science. We just need the correct information and the will to act on it.

In the pages that follow, we'll explore why seed oils are not healthy and why saturated fats are actually a good choice. We'll look at the fats that help us lose weight. We'll share the research regarding various diseases and maladies caused by seed oils. We'll examine each healthy oil and fat in depth, including their smoke points and optimal uses in food preparation, and provide over fifty recipes that incorporate the various fats and oils we recommend. And we'll help you clean out your pantry, select the best oils and fats, and guide you on your road to better health.

CHAPTER 1
Liquid Lies: The Seed Oil Scandal

What if nearly everything you've been told about vegetable oils (a.k.a. seed oils) and animal fats was not true? Your mother believed vegetable oils were a healthy choice. Your teachers. Your doctor. Even the government, scientists, and researchers. They all said the same thing. There were a few dissenting voices, and they were mainly considered the "health nuts." Most people didn't take them seriously. For decades, a large bottle of vegetable oil was a staple in many kitchens. It was affordable, widely available, and considered modern and responsible. Parents cooked with it, grandparents baked with it, and recipes were passed down without question. Whether it was canola oil used for weeknight dinners or Crisco folded into holiday pie crusts, these fats became part of everyday life. No one gave a second thought to the oil in their salad dressings, sauces, and marinades. Not because families were careless—but because when doctors, teachers, scientists, and governments all say something is safe, trust becomes the default.

There's a great awakening now concerning fats and oils. The toxicity of seed oils is trending on TikTok. It's a topic of discussion among young influencers on Instagram. People are questioning the conventional wisdom about fats and oils. Journalists, researchers, doctors, and nutritionists are uncovering a long pattern of misleading practices surrounding these once-celebrated oils. We are witnessing an ancient truth: "Nothing hidden will remain undisclosed." What was once barely questioned is now being brought into the light. Health was never the primary goal in introducing seed oils to the market, which you are about to learn. Profits and convenience drove the engine, and clever marketing mapped the way. They said, "Trust the brand! It's Procter & Gamble's highly respected Crisco, and you don't need to know what's in it. Embrace the modern era of cooking with clean vegetable oils and fluffy white shortening, and leave behind the old, outdated butter and beef tallow."

"Vegetable oil" sounds really wholesome, right? Like something that was pressed from the garden. But seed oils are not manufactured from vegetables—they're made from seeds like soy, rapeseed, sunflower, and corn, using chemical extraction and high-heat processing. The term "vegetable oil" was a marketing concept that sounded natural, wholesome, and healthy, so it was pushed out to the public in attractive marketing campaigns. It was used to soften the stigma of industrial oil that was originally used in machinery, including war machinery. It was the opening act to change a culture—and it was well received. We are exploring the dark side of these oils, exposing what lies behind the rise of industrial seed oils, and what's true and false about conventional teachings on fats and oils.

In the next chapter, we will go into detail on the health problems caused by these oils. As we move forward in this chapter, you'll discover the twists and turns on the underside of the food industry that propelled seed oils into the spotlight of favor—and the surprising truths that were hidden along the way. We'll break down what truly nourishing fats and oils look like, which ones undermine your health, and why it all matters. Consider this your invitation into the real story of oils and fats—a story that just might reshape how you eat, think, and live.

What Are Seed Oils?

Seed oils are the same oils long marketed as "vegetable oils," a name that quietly shifted in the late 2010s as people began asking more questions. Seed oils are extracted from plant seeds like rapeseed (canola), soybean, corn, cottonseed, sunflower, grapeseed, and safflower. These are also known as "the Hateful 8," a term coined by Dr. Cate Shanahan, a board-certified family physical and nutrition researcher. There are a multitude of problems with seed oils. Let's start with the fact that most rapeseeds are genetically modified. Canola was derived from certain rapeseed cultivars. The name canola was established to address the obvious drawbacks of the plant's name. The human body was never designed to thrive on foods engineered in a laboratory.

The ultra-processing plant seeds undergo in the production of oil renders the final product toxic. Such oils are also mostly composed of omega-6 fatty acids, which creates an excess of omega-6 fats and an imbalance of omega-6 to omega-3 fats. This is known to promote inflammation. We have proof these oils can cause a variety of diseases, from heart disease, to cancer, to metabolic disorders, which we'll reference in chapter 2. Of course, these issues don't happen overnight. If you eat seed oil once in a while, you are most likely not going to develop cancer as a result, but if you consistently eat seed oils, your health will decline over time.

There are, however, some seed oils that are healthy, such as flaxseed oil, pumpkin seed oil, hemp seed oil, and sesame seed oil. We know this can get confusing, so to clarify: These seed oils are considered healthy because they are minimally processed and nutrient-rich, and have a favorable balance of healthy omega-3 and omega-6 fats, antioxidants, and anti-inflammatory compounds. They don't cause oxidation in the body. They are typically cold-pressed or expeller-pressed, meaning no chemical solvents or high heat are used, so their delicate nutrients and flavor are preserved. Healthy seed oils provide beneficial fats and phytonutrients that support heart, brain, and cellular health, whereas heavily processed seed oils contribute to oxidative stress and metabolic imbalance. It's important to know that not all seed oils are toxic, so here is a graphic to make it easy to understand.

TOXIC SEED OILS VS. HEALTHY SEED OILS

Toxic Seed oils	Healthy Seed Oils
Canola oil	Black cumin seed oil
Corn oil	Chia seed oil
Cottonseed oil	Flaxseed oil
Grapeseed oil	Hemp seed oil
Peanut oil	Pumpkin seed oil
Rapeseed oil	Sesame seed oil
Rice bran oil	
Safflower oil	
Soybean oil	
Sunflower oil	

The Heart-Healthy Myth

The heart-healthy myth most of us were told for decades was this: "Fat—especially saturated fat—causes heart disease, so eat low-fat foods and replace fat with grains and vegetable oils."

This belief didn't just circulate in magazines or television ads—it was institutionalized.

Beginning in the late 1970s and early 1980s, this idea shaped national dietary guidelines and eventually became visually codified in one of the most influential nutrition graphics of all time: the food pyramid. At the base of the pyramid—the location of foods that were meant to be eaten most often—sat grains and carbohydrates. Bread, cereal, pasta, and rice were encouraged at six to eleven servings per day, while fats were pushed to the very top, labeled something to "use sparingly." Butter, eggs, and red meat were portrayed as dietary threats rather than foundational foods.

This model dominated school lunches, hospital menus, military food programs, and public health messaging for decades. Entire generations were raised to believe that a heart-healthy diet meant low-fat, high-carbohydrate, with vegetable oils positioned as a modern, responsible replacement for traditional animal fats and oils, such as coconut oil.

What We Were Taught

- Butter, eggs, and red meat were harmful
- Low-fat, low-cholesterol diets protected the heart
- Fat should be replaced with carbohydrates
- Vegetable and seed oils were "heart-healthy"
- Calories mattered more than food quality

This framework shaped eating habits well into the twenty-first century, even as rates of obesity, diabetes, and heart disease continued to rise. In recent years, this narrative has begun to unravel. Researchers, clinicians, and independent scientists have revisited the original studies that fueled fat-phobia and found serious methodological flaws, selective data use, and evidence of conflicts of interest. At the same time, real-world outcomes told a different story: As fat intake declined and carbohydrate consumption rose, chronic disease exploded.

By the 2020s, the conversation began to change. Public trust in ultra-processed foods started to erode. Blood sugar regulation, inflammation, and metabolic health entered the spotlight. Long-standing assumptions were questioned—not just by fringe voices, but by mainstream researchers and policymakers.

In January 2026, the US Department of Health and Human Services, the FDA, and the Department of Agriculture under the leadership of Robert F. Kennedy Jr. as Secretary of Health and Human Services, unveiled a new set of Dietary Guidelines for Americans, 2025–2030, described as the most significant reset of federal nutrition policy in decades. These updated guidelines were paired with a reimagined food pyramid that essentially flips the traditional model on its head, prioritizing high-quality protein, healthy fats, vegetables, fruits, whole foods, and significantly reduced reliance on refined carbohydrates, added sugar, and ultra-processed foods—a stark contrast to the six-to-eleven servings of grains encouraged for years in the old model.

Rather than emphasizing avoiding all fats, the new guidance places natural, nutrient-dense fats back into the center of nutrition, supports whole-food sources of protein, and calls for a dramatic reduction in highly processed foods. This represents a fundamental shift in federal dietary messaging—one that acknowledges many of the assumptions behind past guidelines were flawed and that prioritizing real food is essential for reversing America's chronic disease epidemic.

This moment marks a historic turning point in public health guidance. For the first time in generations, federal leadership is openly acknowledging that the low-fat, high-carbohydrate experiment failed to deliver the health outcomes it promised—and that returning to real food will be essential to reversing the modern chronic disease epidemic.

What We Now Know

- Ultra-processed carbohydrates and added sugars drive inflammation and insulin resistance
- Low-fat diets often increase sugar intake, worsening heart risk
- Industrial seed oils, especially when refined and overheated, contribute to oxidative stress
- Whole, natural fats—such as olive oil, avocado, eggs, and grass-fed butter—are not inherently harmful when eaten in real-food form
- Heart disease risk is more closely tied to metabolic dysfunction and chronic inflammation than to natural dietary fat

The Real Foundation of Heart Health

- Whole, minimally processed foods
- Natural fats in their traditional forms
- Clean, adequate protein
- Antioxidant-rich plants
- Minimal sugar and ultra-processed foods
- Sleep, stress management, and lifestyle matter

In simple terms, we weren't taught how to nourish the heart. We were taught how to avoid fat. And in avoiding fat, many people unknowingly replaced it with processed carbohydrates, refined sugars, and industrial oils—a shift that helped fuel the modern chronic disease epidemic.

Fat was never the enemy—yet one of the greatest casualties of the low-fat era was our understanding of how deeply the body depends on healthy fats to heal, regulate, and thrive. Fat is not just fuel; it is structural. The brain is composed of nearly 60 percent fat, and the nervous system relies on fat to insulate nerves, transmit signals, and maintain emotional and cognitive stability. When healthy fats are removed—or replaced with damaged, industrial ones—the body doesn't simply adapt. It destabilizes. Anxiety, brain fog, mood swings, poor focus, hormonal disruption, skin issues, and chronic fatigue are often not signs of weakness but signs of nutritional deprivation.

This became unmistakably clear through clinical experience and personal healing work, explored more deeply later in this book. One of the most effective strategies for calming anxiety and restoring nervous system balance is replenishing healthy fats—particularly omega-3 fatty acids. Years ago, after Liana's blood work revealed a significant omega-3 deficiency, increasing intake through both a high-quality omega-3 supplement and whole-food sources such as wild salmon, walnuts, and hemp seed produced noticeable changes within just three days. Nervous system stability improved. Brain function sharpened. Focus returned. This is not uncommon. The body responds quickly when it is finally given what it has been missing.

We will explore the science behind this in greater depth in later chapters, including how different fats affect the brain, hormones, inflammation, and metabolic health. For now, it's important to understand this foundational truth: the human body was never designed to function without fat. It was designed to be nourished by the right kinds of fat—fats that come from nature, not factories. The tragedy is not that we were told to avoid fat. It's that we were told to fear it—and in doing so, many people unknowingly starved their bodies of one of the most essential nutrients for healing and survival.

This lipid hypothesis was a long-standing theory that shaped modern nutrition policy—and much fear around fat emerged in this very specific historical moment. In the post–World War II era, particularly throughout the 1950s, the United States saw a noticeable rise in reported heart attacks among middle-aged men. Sudden cardiac events appeared to be increasing, and the public—along with physicians and policymakers—was desperate for answers. Something had clearly changed in modern life, and many wanted a single, identifiable cause.

It was within this context that the influential scientist Ancel Keys began studying potential links between diet and heart disease. His attention focused on saturated fat and cholesterol, leading him to propose what became known as the lipid hypothesis—the idea that dietary saturated fat raises blood cholesterol, which in turn causes heart disease. Although his work was based on limited, selective data and sparked controversy at the time, it gained traction because it offered a clear, simple explanation during a period of widespread fear and uncertainty.

Major institutions quickly embraced the theory. The American Heart Association endorsed low-fat dietary guidance, and government agencies followed suit. Once institutionalized, the hypothesis reshaped public nutrition policy almost overnight. Butter and other traditional animal fats fell out of favor, replaced by margarine and newly promoted industrial vegetable oils. Coconut oil, despite its long history of use in traditional cultures, was portrayed as dangerous simply because it contained saturated fat. Food manufacturers seized the opportunity, reformulating products to be low-fat and high-carbohydrate, marketing them as modern and heart-healthy.

What was largely overlooked, however, were other major lifestyle changes occurring at the same time. As physician and nutrition researcher Cate Shanahan has pointed out in her work, cigarette smoking was heavily promoted and widely normalized during this era, including by physicians and advertisers. Smoking rates were extremely high, stress levels were rising, and ultra-processed foods were becoming more common—yet these factors were largely ignored in favor of blaming saturated fat alone.

By focusing narrowly on fat, the lipid hypothesis offered a convenient villain while diverting attention away from other powerful contributors to cardiovascular disease.

Despite its shaky foundation, the saturated fat/cholesterol narrative became the prevailing explanation for the sudden change in American health. Once embedded in medical education, government guidelines, and food manufacturing, it proved remarkably difficult to undo. We discuss this more in The Cholesterol Myth in chapter 3.

During World War II, supplies of coconut oil were cut off when the Japanese occupied most of the Philippines and the South Pacific. Seed oil manufacturers stepped up production and took their place, filling the resulting gap in the marketplace. Vegetable oil sales soared as seed oil companies saw a significant opportunity to steal the market. They paid for slick marketing campaigns, funded research, and influenced the influencers of those times. They paid for cookbooks to be published with seed oils to make them look appealing and show people how to use them. As noted in *The Coconut Diet: The Secret Ingredient That Helps You Lose Weight While You Eat Your Favorite Foods*, Cherie writes, "In short, the industry had an oil boom. When the war ended, the manufacturers weren't going to let go of the market they controlled."[1]

Behind the health claims and marketing hype was a potent economic engine. Government support and aid for popular crops such as cottonseed, linseed, corn, and soybeans, the primary sources of these oils, underpinned these health claims. The oils were artificially cheap due to subsidies. This encouraged mass production. Companies seeking savings used them extensively in processed foods. Big food corporations had financial reasons to promote them, and few stop signs appeared on the road to nutrition advice. There were very few influential voices that raised doubts about the safety of seed oils or brought up the common-sense question: What actually changed in the American diet around the time that heart disease increased exponentially? The result: a food paradigm built on rancid, low-quality, toxic oils, with a false narrative that they were heart-healthy—and a population increasingly afflicted by chronic inflammation, obesity, diabetes, cancer, heart disease, and metabolic disorders.

Nina Teicholz, in *The Big Fat Surprise*, says, "In retrospect, it is perplexing why scientists did not question the assumption that entirely newfangled foodstuffs could restore a population to good health. How could it be that a healthy diet would depend upon these just-invented foods, such as milk 'filled' with soybean oil?"[2]

We were told to "trust the science." But what science were we trusting? Along with seed oils for heart health (the myth), we were encouraged to smoke cigarettes, particularly Camels. It was 1946, and the R. J. Reynolds Tobacco Company launched an advertising campaign for its popular cigarette. Reynolds created the catchy slogan, "More Doctors Smoke Camels Than Any Other Cigarette!" This line was used in their advertising for the next six years. Doctors claimed Camels soothed throats and aided digestion. But smoking created lesions in blood vessels that caused atherosclerotic plaque, which is a buildup of fats and cholesterol. It joined forces with seed oils that did the same thing, along with sugar, which was promoted to replace fat. Then, in the 1950s, breastfeeding became outdated, and baby formula was promoted as a healthier, more modern alternative, driven by marketing and medical endorsements. Baby formula was considered more consistent and predictable than a mother's milk. Sadly, the formula contained seed oils (sunflower, canola, and soy) and still does to this day.[3] It wasn't until the 1970s and 1980s that the pendulum swung back to mother's milk, which was determined to be best for immunity and overall health due to its antibodies. Then came the egg scare of the 1970s, when the public was advised to avoid eggs, or rather egg yolks, because they contained cholesterol and were linked to high blood cholesterol, which was part of the plaque found in arteries (but so were triglycerides and fatty acids). For nearly two decades, the nation choked down egg whites and threw away the more nutritious yolks. The message changed in 1999, when a study published in *JAMA*, a leading medical journal, found no link between egg consumption and cardiovascular disease risk.[4] But they discovered something else—eating egg whites without the yolk can bind biotin (vitamin B7) and cause a condition known as egg white injury due to biotin deficiency.

Big Fat Lies

False information with good intentions? Misrepresentation of facts? Manipulation of data to promote an honored theory? It's all still a lie, no matter how you phrase it. If you repeat a lie often enough, it starts to sound like the truth. It becomes familiar, and everyone repeats it. If you support that lie, backed by billion-dollar industries, government funding, prestigious organizations with gala fundraisers, flawed research, nutritional dogma, lobbying, and slick advertising campaigns, it becomes gospel. We have been fed false information for decades—a steady stream of misinformation that has been ingrained in our brains until it became accepted and defended by nearly everyone. That was until a new breed of truth seekers emerged, and finally, with Robert F. Kennedy Jr., as the Make America Healthy Again (MAHA) leader, voiced the truth: Seed oils are not heart-healthy, as we've been told for decades. They are, in fact, toxic and poisonous. RFK Jr posted on X in October 2024, saying how seed oils have "unknowingly poisoned" Americans and that they are "one of the driving causes of the obesity epidemic."

The Lipid Theory Trap

Once something gets carved into the halls of nutrition science, it isn't easy to introduce a new paradigm. Inherently, people tend to dislike change. Couple that with professional pride that says, "I couldn't possibly have been wrong all these years about vegetable oils. There's no way I was teaching and promoting something false," and you'll find a well-defended fortress of thought with all the science soldiers at the gates protecting their territory—alongside powerful investors with deep financial stakes in the seed oil business.

Recently, Cherie looked at a skillet that she'd used to cook meat in beef tallow. It was soaking in the sink with little globs of white fat floating in the water. She cringed as she looked at that fat. She thought, "We have been so brainwashed to view animal fat negatively that my innate reaction is still adverse in the face of the truths I've learned in recent years." She had to laugh. She was living what she was writing about. Old lies don't die easily, even in the presence of truth.

Nina Teicholz, in *The Big Fat Surprise*, says:

> One of the twentieth century's most revered nutrition scientists, organic chemist David Kritchevsky, discovered this [resistance] thirty years ago when, on a panel for the National Academy of Sciences, he suggested loosening the restrictions on dietary fat. "We were jumped on!" he told me. "People would spit on us!" It's hard to imagine now the heat of passion. It was just like we had desecrated the American flag. They were so angry that we were going against the suggestions of the American Heart Association and the National Institutes of Health. This kind of opposition met all experts who criticized the prevailing view on dietary fat, effectively silencing all opposition. Researchers who persisted in their challenges found themselves cut off from grants, unable to rise in their professional societies, without invitations to serve on expert panels, and at a loss to find scientific journals that would publish their papers. Their influence was extinguished, and their viewpoints lost.[5]

Even Ancel Keys, the pioneering American physiologist and the father of the lipid theory, who proposed the diet-heart hypothesis linking dietary saturated fat intake to cardiovascular disease, later changed his mind before his death. As research evolved, he began to reconsider this link between saturated fat and heart disease.[6] But Keyes was not listened to at this point. The American Heart Association (AHA), which promoted vegetable oils as "heart healthy," had a major undisclosed conflict of interest and was significantly funded by Procter & Gamble, the maker of Crisco (short for "crystallized cottonseed oil"). This influence transformed the AHA from a regional organization into a national powerhouse and led to the dissemination of biased health guidance. They helped shape public policy and "write the rules of nutrition."[7, 8]

Do you want to see firsthand just how ingrained seed oil groupthink is today? Google "Are seed oils healthy?" or "Are polyunsaturated fats unhealthy?" You'll mostly get the same responses about vegetable oils and omega-6 fatty acids on every website. They all say nearly the same thing—they are heart-healthy and lower LDL. Ask ChatGPT. It's programmed with the same information. Those bots have the same story! Even Chelsea Clinton blamed "Big Olive Oil" on her podcast for demeaning seed oils.

Who will champion the cause? Where have the voices been in the weeds of misinformation? They are few, and the establishment, influenced by corporate interests, mostly drowned them out. But the voices of influencers on social media are growing louder and more prominent each day. And RFK Jr. is a well-known champion leading the charge. Still, we need many other voices to join us in our goal to spread the truth across America. The truth-tellers cannot move forward most effectively without you. You can discuss fats and oils with your neighbor, talk to your coworkers, and bring it up with family members. With truth crisscrossing America at the grassroots level, we can win this war of words.

We achieved a big win concerning margarine. Margarine's decline has been steady since the 1990s, primarily due to the public's increasing awareness of the health effects of the trans fats it contains. Many of us wrote about it and informed our followers of its dangers. Look around any grocery store shelf today, and you won't see a large selection of margarine, whereas it used to dominate the shelves. We can do it again with seed oils.

The Twelve Red Flags of Seed Oils

1. Ultra-processed and not found in nature
    - Seed oils are industrial products, not traditional foods.
    - Most seeds are derived from genetically modified seeds (unless organic) and require extensive processing that does not occur naturally. (The top four are: soybean, corn, cottonseed, and canola.)

2. Extracted using high heat and chemical solvents
    - Commonly processed with high temperatures, pressure, and chemical solvents such as hexane.
    - This process can create toxic by-products before the oil even reaches the shelf.
3. High in unstable polyunsaturated fats (PUFAs)
    - Seed oils are rich in polyunsaturated fatty acids with fragile double bonds.
    - These bonds are easily damaged by heat, light, and oxygen, making the oils highly unstable.
4. Oxidation and rancidity
    - Due to their instability, seed oils oxidize easily during processing, storage, and cooking.
    - Oxidized oils generate harmful compounds linked to oxidative stress and cellular damage. Oxidative stress plays a significant role in the development of cancer through DNA damage and chronic inflammation.
5. Widely used in restaurant cooking and processed foods
    - Seed oils are the primary fats used in 99 percent of restaurants, fast-food, and packaged foods because they are cheap and shelf-stable.
    - This leads to chronic, unintentional overconsumption.
6. Excess omega-6 fatty acids
    - Seed oils are extremely high in omega-6 fatty acids, particularly linoleic acid.
    - Significant intake contributes to an imbalanced ratio of omega-6 to omega-3.
7. Inflammation and immune disruption
    - Excess omega-6 intake is associated with inflammatory signaling pathways.
    - Chronic inflammation is a known contributor to many long-term diseases.

8. Formation of toxic compounds when heated
    - When used for frying or high-heat cooking, seed oils can break down into aldehydes and other toxic compounds.
    - These compounds have been linked in studies to DNA damage and metabolic stress.
9. Associations with chronic disease
10. Oxidative stress and chronic inflammation from excessive seed oil intake have been linked in research to a host of conditions, including cancer (via inflammatory and oxidative mechanisms), cardiovascular disease, obesity, insulin resistance, and neurodegenerative conditions such as dementia and Alzheimer's disease (associative and mechanistic evidence, not claims of direct causation)
11. Displacement of traditional, stable fats
    - The rise of seed oils has largely replaced traditional fats like butter, olive oil, coconut oil, and animal fats that humans consumed for thousands of years.
12. Loss of natural antioxidants
    - Industrial refining strips seed oils of naturally occurring antioxidants, such as vitamin E and polyphenols.
    - Without these protective compounds, seed oils are far more susceptible to oxidation both on the shelf and in the body.
13. Lack of evolutionary precedent
    - Humans did not consume concentrated seed oils for thousands of years.
    - Their widespread use began only in the last century, making them an evolutionary mismatch for human metabolism.

We need to eat real foods from nature that we thrived on for thousands of years. Are industrially processed foods and seed oils really better for you? Nope, just better for their bottom line. The food of the future, if we are to reverse this epidemic of disease, is real food in its whole form as God made it, minimally processed with the nutrients intact.

WHERE YOU'LL FIND SEED OILS

Seed oils are mostly found in these eight foods:

1. Salad dressings
2. Mayonnaise
3. Sauces and marinades
4. Packaged snacks
5. Protein bars
6. Dairy-free products
7. Restaurant foods
8. Infant formula

Found Especially In:

- Restaurant food
    - Fryers (French fries, fried chicken, chips)
    - Sautéed vegetables, meats, and seafood
    - Salad dressings and sauces made in-house
    - "Grilled" foods brushed with oil
- Fast food
    - Fries, nuggets, burgers, wraps
    - Breakfast sandwiches
    - Anything fried or cooked on a flattop
- Packaged and ultra-processed foods
    - Chips, crackers, pretzels
    - Cookies, cakes, muffins, pastries
    - Protein bars, granola bars, energy bars
    - Breakfast cereals and granola
    - Frozen meals and pizzas
- "Health" foods (often surprising)
    - Gluten-free snacks and crackers
    - Vegan and plant-based products
    - Protein powders and meal replacements

    - Nut butters and seed butters
    - Dairy-free yogurts and creamers
- Condiments and sauces
    - Salad dressings (even "olive oil" blends)
    - Mayonnaise
    - Ketchup, barbecue sauce, marinades
    - Pesto, aioli, flavored spreads
- Baked goods
    - Store-bought bread and tortillas
    - Bagels, buns, wraps
    - Piecrusts, cookies, brownies
    - "Low-fat" or shelf-stable baked items
- Cooking oils at home
    - Vegetable oil
    - Canola (rapeseed) oil
    - Corn oil
    - Soybean oil
    - Sunflower or safflower oil
    - Grapeseed oil
    - Rice bran oil
- Prepared foods
    - Deli items
    - Rotisserie chicken
    - Pre-marinated meats
    - Ready-to-eat salads
    - Meal kits
- Baby and children's foods
    - Infant formula
    - Baby food pouches
    - Toddler snacks
    - Kids' cereals and bars

(continued . . .)

- Ethnic and specialty foods
  - Takeout (Asian, Mexican, Mediterranean)
  - Premade hummus and dips
  - Store-bought flatbreads and wraps
- Even products with these labels can contain seed oils
  - "Organic"
  - "Natural"
  - "Heart-healthy"
  - "Plant-based"
  - "Cholesterol-free"

Seed oils are often listed in small print under names like non-GMO canola oil, soybean oil, sunflower oil, safflower oil, vegetable oil, or blends.

"Blends" and Vague Terms

- Vegetable oil blend
- Plant-based oil blend
- Cooking oil
- Frying oil
- Proprietary oil blend

(These almost always include one or more seed oils.)

Processed-Fat Derivatives

- Margarine
- Shortening
- Hydrogenated oil
- Partially hydrogenated oil
- Interesterified fats

Ingredients That Often Signal Seed Oils Are Present

- Lecithin (soy lecithin, sunflower lecithin)

- Mono- and diglycerides
- Emulsifiers (often derived from seed oils)

"Health-Washed" Names

- Heart-healthy oil
- Cholesterol-free oil
- Light oil
- Pure vegetable oil
- Omega-6 oil

If the label says "vegetable oil" and doesn't specify olive oil, avocado oil, or coconut oil, it is almost always a seed oil.

The Dark History of Seed Oils

Before the early 1900s, people used animal fats, such as tallow and butter, for nearly everything. In the late 1800s, as cotton production exploded across the United States following the Civil War, vast quantities of cottonseed—once considered toxic waste—began piling up and rotting. Farmers had grown cotton for its fiber, not its seed, and the by-product posed a growing disposal problem. Chemists and manufacturers soon discovered that oil could be extracted from cottonseed and refined through a bleaching and deodorizing process, neutralizing its toxins and making it usable for industrial purposes such as soaps, lubricants, and lamps. What began as an industrial solution eventually became a commercial opportunity. By the early twentieth century, companies sought to incorporate cottonseed oil into the food supply, despite public resistance and early food adulteration scandals.

Initial attempts to mill the seeds yielded a dark, smelly oil used in industrial dyes, roofing tar, machinery, and explosives, and then in ships and aircraft during World War II. After the war, manufacturers were left with an abundance of industrial seed oils and large-scale processing infrastructure originally used for machinery lubricants, soaps, and wartime materials. Rather than discard it, they repurposed it for the food supply. These oils were cheap to produce, shelf-stable, and highly profitable—but they weren't naturally appealing to consumers. To make them acceptable, and even desirable, a massive marketing campaign was launched to rebrand industrial oils as modern, heart-healthy "vegetable oils" for the American kitchen.

Chemist David Wesson emerged in the late nineteenth century and introduced industrial processing techniques, including bleaching and deodorizing. This produced a transparent, tasteless, and neutral-smelling oil that was appealing to consumers. Soon, companies began selling cottonseed oil and also mixing it with animal fats, such as lard.

Cottonseed oil was the first to be restructured. In 1911, Procter & Gamble figured out how to hydrogenate it into a solid fat, marketing Crisco, a brand of vegetable shortening that didn't spoil and didn't need refrigeration. It was developed through a process used to produce hardened soap. Crisco was advertised as cleaner, more modern, and healthier than lard or butter. That defined a new beginning in food science and edible oils.

As extraction methods improved, other seed oils emerged, including soybean, corn, canola, safflower, and sunflower oils. These oils were not pressed like olive oil, but extracted with high heat and solvents such as hexane, then bleached and deodorized to mask rancid flavors and smells. Seed oils were widely available by mid-century and offered the perfect solution for food corporations. They were considered ideal replacements for the fats and oils currently used; they were inexpensive, easy to store, and well-suited for processed foods. America embraced them with open arms, and the modern era of cooking and food manufacturing flourished.

Housewives all across America welcomed vegetable oils; after all, who doesn't want vegetable products? Cookbooks were compiled featuring recipes that used the new oil. A new era of cooking began in the American kitchen. But something else showed up—myocardial infarction. Obesity rates rose. In the mid-twentieth century, diabetes became an epidemic. Metabolic syndrome was recognized for the first time. Amid the alarming decline in health, almost no one asked what had changed. They pointed to butter, beef tallow, and coconut oil and said that the saturated fat in these products had caused the rapid escalation of these health problems. What happened to the scientists and researchers? No one said "Wait—we've been consuming these fats for centuries without an increase in diseases. Why would animal fats or coconut oil suddenly make us fat and clog our arteries?" Modern civilization was facing diseases not previously seen, at such alarming rates that it drew the attention of doctors, scientists, and even the government. Everyone wanted answers.

Industrial Processing of Seed Oils

The refining, bleaching, and deodorizing of seed oils oxidize their fatty acids, and the use of toxic chemicals can generate toxins that promote oxidative stress. Also, refining removes most of the antioxidants.

According to Eric Decker, a professor at the University of Massachusetts Amherst, there are five significant steps in processing industrial seed oils:

- **Degumming.** This process removes phospholipids, which can cloud the oil and impart off-flavors, thereby reducing its stability. Oil processors use citric acid, which is the same thing you'll find in citrus fruit, to encourage the phospholipids to leave the oil.
- **Neutralization.** That takes away free fatty acids, which can cause off-flavors and shorten an oil's shelf life. To achieve that, manufacturers mix the oil with sodium hydroxide to separate the fatty acids from the rest of the oil. Decker says, "They recapture those fatty acids and sell them to the soap industry."
- **Bleaching.** The goal of bleaching is to achieve a very color-consistent product, but also get rid of chlorophyll," Decker says, referring to the green pigment in plants that will speed up the onset of rancidity. The oil is mixed with a filter aid, typically bentonite clay, which binds to the pigments, allowing them to be filtered out.
- **Deodorization.** This process adds steam to the oil, holds it under vacuum, and then releases the steam. That removes any off-aromas that could be in the oil.

- **Chemical extraction.** This process uses hexane because the manufacturer wants to recover 100 percent of the oil from the seed. Cold pressing leaves much of the oil in the pomace, the solid material left over after pressing. Hexane is the most effective way to strip it all out. The European Food Safety Authority is reviewing the use of hexane in food manufacturing.[9, 10]

The truth is that it's hard to remove all the stuff you don't want, like gums, off-flavors, and compounds that can make seed oils go rancid, along with preserving the nutrients you do want, like antioxidants. And then there are the chemicals, such as hexane. Numerous health professionals and educators say, "Don't worry about the hexane. Most of it is removed, and what's left evaporates when you heat it." Is that supposed to make us feel good about traces of harmful chemicals like hexane left in our cooking oil? Hexane is a neurotoxic chemical that can cause potential harm to the nervous system. The US Environmental Protection Agency is considering alternatives to hexane due to its toxicity.[11]

Here's the real question worth asking: How could heavily refined, industrial seed oils that were never intended as food in the first place possibly be good for us? These oils are produced through complex factory processes that use chemicals and methods far removed from anything natural or nourishing. They're newcomers—barely a blip in human history—compared to traditional fats like butter churned from cream or oils such as coconut, extracted through simple, time-honored techniques. And it's no coincidence that as seed oils entered our food supply, our nation's health began to unravel at a startling pace.

How Canola Oil Was Created

Canola oil did not exist in the human diet for most of history. It is a relatively modern invention, developed in the twentieth century through agricultural intervention and industrial processing. The oil began as rapeseed, a naturally occurring plant in the mustard family. For centuries, rapeseed oil was not commonly consumed as food. It contained naturally high levels of erucic acid and bitter compounds, making it unsuitable for regular dietary use. Instead, it was primarily used for industrial purposes such as lamp oil and mechanical lubrication.

In the 1970s, plant breeders in Canada selectively bred rapeseed to reduce its erucic acid content and bitterness. This newly altered crop was renamed canola, short for Canadian Oil, Low Acid. The goal was to create an inexpensive, shelf-stable oil that could be widely consumed and easily incorporated into the modern food supply. Although the early development of canola involved selective breeding rather than genetic engineering, it was still a deliberate human alteration of a plant that had not traditionally been eaten in this form. Over time, canola became one of the most widely used oils in the world.

Modern canola oil is not extracted through simple, traditional methods. Instead, the seeds undergo an industrial process that includes crushing, high-heat treatment, chemical solvent extraction, bleaching, and deodorization. These steps are necessary to produce a neutral-tasting, clear oil with a long shelf life, but they also significantly alter the oil from its original state.

Today, most of the global canola supply is also genetically modified, primarily to withstand herbicides and increase crop yields. By the time canola oil reaches supermarket shelves, it is far removed from the original seed from which it came. The distinction matters. Rapeseed is a naturally occurring plant, but canola oil is a modern, industrial product—designed for efficiency, affordability, and mass consumption rather than traditional nourishment. Ironically, it gained a reputation as the healthiest cooking oil. Restaurants proudly acknowledged that their recipes were made with canola oil. And the public believed they were preparing at-home meals with the best vegetable oil available.

Understanding how canola oil is made helps explain why it differs so profoundly from fats humans have relied on for generations, such as olive oil, butter, and animal fats, which were traditionally consumed in forms much closer to their natural state.

This is where the confusion deepens. It doesn't matter if a bottle of canola oil is marketed as "organic" or "non-GMO"—it remains a highly refined industrial oil that was literally created by scientists in laboratories, not something that exists in nature. When a food that never existed naturally is labeled "organic" or "non-GMO," it raises a critical question: What do those labels really mean? This is a false sense of safety that leads well-intentioned consumers to trust products that are still fundamentally industrial and far from "organic" or "non-genetically modified."

We Can Change America

Are you tired of being lied to and poisoned with toxic seed oils, all because of money and greed? It's time to vote with your dollars. Avoid purchasing products that contain seed oils. Don't cook with them. Choose restaurants that use healthy fats and oils in their dishes. (See chapter 6 for restaurant guides.) Get the word out on social media. Tell your friends and family. Make your voice heard. And don't buy into groupthink about the benefits of seed oils, even when it comes from a well-respected organization or individual. How many lives could be saved because of this truth? Join the movement—NO MORE SEED OILS IN AMERICA! As RFK Jr. would say, "It's time to make frying tallow again." After all, the world-famous McDonald's French fries, introduced in 1949, were originally cooked in beef tallow.

CHAPTER 2

Seed Oils Cause Anxiety, Depression, Cancer, Alzheimer's, Dementia, and Worse

This chapter explores a growing scientific debate that is only now entering mainstream nutrition conversations. The explosion of seed oils in the modern food supply is implicated not only in inflammation and metabolic disease, heart disease, and cancer, but increasingly in mental health disorders, cognitive decline, and yes, even aggression.

This is not fringe theory. This is biochemistry.

Of course, not everyone who has ever consumed seed oils will experience these outcomes, but evidence suggests that greater and more prolonged exposure—especially to oxidized seed oils—correlates with higher risk of inflammation-driven mental, neurological, and cancer-related diseases. And we are about to present you with a ton of science to back it up.

After reading this chapter and examining the science, you will see that it is clear: seed oils are an assault on both brain health and overall well-being.

The Brain Is Made of Fat—And It Cares Which Kind

The human brain is nearly 60 percent fat by dry weight. That fat is not interchangeable. Healthy brains evolved on omega-3–rich fats from flaxseed oil, along with small amounts present in olive oil, wild seafood, and pastured animals. Other important fats for the brain include medium-chain triglycerides in coconut oil and full-fat dairy, plus monounsaturated fats in olive oil and avocados. Today, those fats have been displaced by industrial seed oils that are:

- chemically extracted
- heat- and solvent-processed
- deodorized, and
- highly unstable.

These oils flood the brain and body with excess omega-6 linoleic acid, which is highly unstable and prone to oxidation. When heated, processed, or stored, seed oils readily break down into toxic lipid peroxides and aldehydes, triggering oxidative stress at the cellular level. This oxidative damage fuels chronic inflammation while simultaneously crowding out omega-3 fats like DHA and EPA—the very fats required for emotional regulation, memory, hormonal balance, and resilience to stress.

Worse still, oxidized seed oils impair mitochondrial function, disrupting the cell's ability to produce clean energy, and contribute to insulin resistance, blood-brain barrier dysfunction, and increased gut permeability. Over time, this biochemical chaos places the nervous system in a constant state of threat, making the brain more vulnerable to anxiety, mood disorders, cognitive decline, and inflammatory diseases.

If we look to our ancestors and indigenous peoples who never consumed industrial seed oils, do you think they faced widespread issues like dementia, Alzheimer's, or the chronic diseases common in modern society? If we apply a bit of common sense, it seems wise to stick with the foods and natural oils that our Creator provided—foods our bodies were designed to digest and metabolize.

While we cannot go back in time to measure Alzheimer's, dementia, heart disease, or cancer rates in ancestral populations with modern diagnostic tools, anthropological and nutritional research suggests that traditional, whole-food diets—free from industrial seed oils—were associated with remarkably low rates of chronic Western diseases. For instance, the Tsimané people of the Bolivian Amazon, who live a traditional lifestyle without industrial seed oils, exhibit one of the lowest recorded rates of dementia in the world—around 1 percent in older adults, compared with roughly 11 percent in the United States.[1] They also have exceptionally low rates of heart disease, reinforcing the connection between diet, metabolic health, and chronic disease outcomes.

Modern nutritional research supports this pattern. Studies of Mediterranean-style diets, which emphasize unprocessed foods and traditional fats such as olive oil, consistently demonstrate reduced risk of cardiovascular disease, cancer, and cognitive decline.[2] Similarly, the Adventist Health Studies show that populations adhering to whole-food, minimally processed diets experience lower rates of chronic disease, including cancer, compared with the general population.[3] Large cohort studies like EPIC (European Prospective Investigation into Cancer and Nutrition) further corroborate that diet quality strongly influences cancer and disease risk.[4]

Even research on neurodegenerative diseases highlights the impact of diet. Western dietary patterns—high in processed foods, refined carbohydrates, and industrial fats—are associated with increased risk of Alzheimer's and dementia through mechanisms involving insulin resistance, oxidative stress, and chronic inflammation.[5] Taken together, these lines of evidence suggest that diets composed of whole, natural fats and minimally processed foods, like those consumed by our ancestors, supported health in ways that modern diets often do not.

The Science: Why Seed Oils Can Be Damaging to the Brain Itself

1. Oxidative Stress and Toxic By-Products

Seed oils are high in fragile polyunsaturated fats (PUFAs) that easily oxidize, creating compounds that can cause oxidative stress on the brain and nervous system. Polyunsaturated fats themselves are not inherently bad. The problem is the type, amount, and processing—especially modern seed oils. PUFAs, like those in seed oils, are chemically unstable, especially when exposed to heat or processing. This instability produces oxidative by-products, such as aldehydes, which are toxic to cells. These compounds can damage neurons directly and stress mitochondria, the energy factories of cells. Neurons are particularly sensitive to oxidative damage, and chronic exposure can impair brain function.

Animal and human cell studies demonstrate that oxidized seed oils increase markers of cellular stress in brain tissues, compared to more stable fats like olive oil or coconut oil.[6] Chronic oxidative stress accelerates cell aging, inflammation, and neurotransmitter dysfunction, all of which are linked to cognitive decline and mental health disorders.

Not So Heart-Healthy

The notion that PUFAs are best for your heart has some cracks in its foundation. Although these fats can lower LDL cholesterol, that doesn't necessarily translate into a lower risk of heart disease. The Minnesota Coronary Experiment (1968–1973) was a study of nine thousand participants that found replacing saturated fat with polyunsaturated fat lowered cholesterol levels, but it did not reduce mortality; indeed, it may have marginally increased it. Older participants who experienced the greatest lowering of cholesterol died at higher rates.[7] Why? Oxidized PUFAs and their pro-inflammatory derivatives can damage blood vessels, promote plaque growth, and destabilize existing plaques, leading to heart attacks. They could be called silent killers: you usually don't see them or taste them, but they are "burning down your house" with inflammation. RFK Jr., Secretary of Health and Human Services, said, "We are being unknowingly poisoned" by seed oils and urged people to revert to 'traditional' fats such as butter and beef drippings for better health."[8]

"Forget the 'science' that has been drummed into your head for decades," says heart surgeon Dr. Lundell. "The science that saturated fat alone causes heart disease is nonexistent. The science that saturated fat raises blood cholesterol is also very weak. Since we now know that cholesterol is not the cause of heart disease, the concern about saturated fat is even more absurd today."[9]

2. Neuroinflammation

Highly processed seed oils are overwhelmingly rich in linoleic acid (LA), a type of omega-6 polyunsaturated fat. When consumed in excess—especially without sufficient omega-3 intake—LA can drive pro-inflammatory pathways in the brain. The balance between omega-6 and omega-3 fatty acids is critical for neurological health. Traditional diets are estimated to have provided an omega-6 to omega-3 ratio of roughly 1:1 to 4:1, whereas modern Western diets often exceed 15:1. This extreme imbalance has been associated in the scientific literature with increased neuroinflammation, higher rates of depression, and cognitive decline.[10]

Seed oils are particularly problematic because polyunsaturated fats, such as linoleic acid, are chemically unstable and highly prone to oxidation. Research shows that these fats oxidize easily under heat, during processing, and even within the body under metabolic stress, forming reactive lipid by-products that increase oxidative stress—a well-recognized trigger for inflammation in the brain.[11]

Once consumed in excess, linoleic acid is converted into arachidonic acid, which the body uses to produce inflammatory signaling molecules such as prostaglandins and leukotrienes. While these compounds play a role in normal immune responses, chronic overproduction can promote persistent inflammatory signaling, including within neural tissue.[12]

Animal and mechanistic studies further suggest that high linoleic acid intake may increase the brain's vulnerability to neuroinflammation, particularly when omega-3 intake is low. A review published in *Translational Psychiatry* discusses how linoleic acid and its oxidized metabolites can influence neuronal stress pathways, mitochondrial function, and inflammatory responses in the brain.[13]

Compounding the issue, excess omega-6 intake competes directly with omega-3 fats such as DHA and EPA, which are critical structural components of the brain and play a central role in resolving inflammation. DHA supports neurotransmission, protects neurons, and helps maintain mitochondrial energy production. Diets disproportionately high in omega-6 fats have been shown to reduce DHA availability in brain tissue, weakening the brain's ability to regulate inflammation and recover from stress.[14]

What Inflammation in the Brain Can Cause

Neuroinflammation—the activation of immune cells within the brain—has been linked in the scientific literature to disrupted neurotransmitter signaling, impaired mitochondrial energy production, increased blood-brain barrier permeability, and altered stress-response pathways.[15]

Neuroinflammation directly affects key neurotransmitter systems, including serotonin, dopamine, and GABA, which regulate mood, motivation, stress response, sleep, and emotional resilience. Over time, this inflammatory environment may contribute to symptoms such as brain fog, memory issues, anxiety, low mood, headaches, fatigue, sleep disturbances, and reduced stress tolerance, reflecting an over-activated immune response rather than a lack of mental clarity or willpower.[16]

3. Disrupted Neurotransmitter Balance

Excess omega-6 relative to omega-3 doesn't just drive inflammation; it also interferes with neurotransmitter synthesis and function. Serotonin, dopamine, and GABA rely on proper cellular signaling and membrane integrity. Too much omega-6 can alter cell membrane composition, reducing the efficiency of neurotransmitter release and receptor function. Mechanistically, this contributes to mood disorders, anxiety, poor motivation, and disrupted stress responses.[17]

Neurotransmitters are the brain's chemical messengers. When they are disrupted, it can directly affect mood, memory, focus, and cognitive resilience, explaining why excess seed oil consumption may be linked to depression, anxiety, and cognitive decline.

4. Mitochondrial Dysfunction

Since seed oils are rich in PUFAs, they are highly prone to oxidation. When oxidized, they can damage mitochondria, the energy-producing structures in cells. Neurons are highly energy-dependent, so mitochondrial dysfunction can lead to impaired cognition, fatigue, and poor memory. Oxidized PUFAs impair mitochondrial function and increase oxidative stress in neuronal cells.[18]

5. Lipid Peroxidation and Brain Cell Damage

PUFAs in seed oils can undergo lipid peroxidation, producing reactive aldehydes such as 4-HNE, which can damage DNA, proteins, and membranes. Lipid peroxidation is strongly implicated in neurodegenerative diseases, including Alzheimer's and Parkinson's. High dietary omega-6 increases brain lipid peroxidation and cognitive decline in animal models.[19]

6. Microglial Activation

Microglia are the brain's immune cells. Chronic inflammation caused by high omega-6 intake can over-activate microglia, leading to neuronal damage and synaptic loss. This process contributes to cognitive decline, memory loss, and increased risk of dementia. Omega-6 PUFA consumption triggers pro-inflammatory microglial responses.[20]

7. Endocannabinoid System Disruption

Endocannabinoids, which regulate mood, appetite, and stress responses, are synthesized from fatty acids. Excess linoleic acid (omega-6) can alter endocannabinoid signaling. Disrupted signaling has shown to lead to increased anxiety, depression, and impaired stress response. Dietary omega-6/omega-3 imbalance affects endocannabinoid signaling in the brain.[21]

8. Blood-Brain Barrier Integrity

Chronic consumption of oxidized and highly processed PUFAs can impair the blood-brain barrier, allowing toxins and inflammatory molecules to enter the brain. Compromised barrier function is associated with neuroinflammation and neurodegeneration. Dietary lipids affect blood-brain barrier permeability.[22]

9. The Omega-6 and Omega-3 Imbalance

There is compelling evidence that an imbalance of omega-6 fats to omega-3s can lead to various ailments that include:

- **Chronic inflammatory diseases** such as rheumatoid arthritis and inflammatory bowel disease.
- **Life expectancy reduction.** Countries with traditional diets rich in omega-3 show longer life expectancy than those with high omega-6 intake and low in omega-3 intake.
- **Disease risk.** A higher intake of omega-6 fats to omega-3s is associated with a greater risk of dying, particularly of heart disease and cancer.[23]

Omega-6 and omega-3 fatty acids comprise PUFAs. Fish oil, flax, and chia seeds are good sources of omega-3s, while omega-6 fats are abundant in vegetable oils, nuts, and seeds. Omega-6s are essential in small amounts, but the modern diet provides them in excessive quantities. "One tablespoon of corn oil contains 7,280 mg of omega-6; one tablespoon of soybean oil contains 6,940 mg."[24]

The average American consumes twenty to thirty times the amount of omega-6s as they do omega-3s—a ratio that is wildly out of sync with our physical needs. The average person consumes a ratio of about 15:1 omega-6 to omega-3 fats. When you compare this to the ancestral diet, which had a 1:1 to 1:4 ratio, you see how out of balance our modern diet has become. This produces inflammation that leads to chronic disease. "It's like living with a low-grade fever that never seems to break."[25]

Other health issues like diabetes, obesity, and cancer have also been linked to high PUFA intake. One study found that omega-6 fats, specifically linoleic acid, may promote tumor growth in certain cancers by providing fuel for proliferation and inducing inflammation and oxidative stress.[26]

Why are so many people on antidepressants? Taking these prescription medications is a growing trend, especially among young women. There are multiple reasons for depression, but seed oils can be a major contributor. John Stein, Emeritus Professor of Neurosciences at Oxford, says, "If you eat too much corn oil or sunflower oil, the brain is absorbing too much omega-6s, and that effectively forces out omega-3s. I believe the lack of omega-3 is a powerful contributory factor to such problems as increasing mental health issues and other problems, such as dyslexia." Stein says he has replaced sunflower oil and corn oil with olive oil and butter in his kitchen.[27]

Too many omega-6s can hinder brain functioning. In thirteen animal studies, brain composition, pathology, and behavior associated with Alzheimer's disease were influenced by the omega-6-to-omega-3 fatty acid ratio in the diet.[28] It was also reported that "a high serum DGLA, which is an omega-6 polyunsaturated fatty acid, has been associated with obesity, body fat accumulation, a high alanine aminotransferase level, and insulin resistance in Japanese subjects with type 2 diabetes."[29]

10. Disrupted Dopamine Signals Cause Intense Cravings

Excessive consumption of omega-6 fatty acids from seed oils, can increase the appetite for foods rich in carbohydrates and sugars. This is the plight of contemporary people. Most snack foods are high in sugar, sodium, and refined carbohydrates, causing people to over-consume them because of their appealing taste, texture, and addictive ingredients. The result is obesity and insulin resistance. Dr. Lundell says, "There is no escaping the fact that the more we consume prepared and processed foods, the more we trip the inflammation switch little by little each day. The human body cannot process, nor was it designed to consume, foods packed with sugars and soaked in omega-6 oils."[30]

THE REAL COST OF SEED OILS

- Oxidative by-products from unstable PUFAs → neuronal damage
- High omega-6 intake → inflammation in the brain and throughout the body
- Disrupted neurotransmitters → mood and cognitive dysfunction
- Impair mitochondria → less energy for neurons
- Lipid peroxidation → cell and DNA damage
- Over-activate microglia → chronic neuroinflammation
- Disrupted endocannabinoid signaling → mood and stress issues
- Disrupted dopamine signaling → increased appetite and cravings for sugar and carbs
- Compromised blood-brain barrier → increased vulnerability to toxins

Anxiety and Depression

Seed oils are strongly implicated in mood disorders due to their high content of linoleic acid (LA), the dominant omega-6 fatty acid. While the conversation often focuses on total omega-6 intake, what truly matters biologically is the balance between omega-6 and omega-3 fatty acids. Diets high in industrial seed oils dramatically skew this ratio, promoting neuroinflammation and disrupting neurotransmitter signaling. Research supports this: A peer-reviewed analysis found that higher linoleic acid intake was associated with greater odds of psychological distress and depression in adults.[31]

This imbalance can impair serotonin, dopamine, and GABA pathways, which are central to mood regulation, stress response, and motivation. The result is a higher likelihood of experiencing anxiety, low mood, and emotional instability, especially in populations consuming modern Western diets rich in seed oils.

Omega-3 Deficiency Is One of the Most Common Nutritional Drivers of Anxiety

DHA (docosahexaenoic acid) is a primary structural component of the brain and cerebral cortex. Low DHA levels are associated with:

- generalized anxiety
- major depressive disorder
- anxiety-like behavior
- impaired cognition

Multiple studies show that DHA supplementation has anxiolytic (anxiety-reducing) effects, while deficiency correlates with worsened mental health outcomes. In Liana's own case, within three days of deliberately increasing omega-3 intake, her nervous system stabilized. She felt calmer, more emotionally regulated, and less reactive. Nothing else changed. The food did.

When Liana wrote her book *Anxiety Free with Food*, she researched the top foods proven to contribute to anxiety, and the results were striking. Refined sugar ranked first, and trans fats—found in fried foods, fast foods, conventional nondairy creamers, and hydrogenated oils—came in second. These are the "bad fats" that have the most direct impact on mood and mental health. Trans fats are largely man-made, created when liquid seed (vegetable) oils are partially hydrogenated—a process that turns them into solid or semisolid fats at room temperature. Partial hydrogenation produces the harmful trans fats that should be avoided entirely.

Trans fats became common in the 1950s and are found in margarine, snack foods, chips, packaged baked goods, shortening, and oils used to fry fast food. Their negative impact on public health is so significant that the World Health Organization released a global initiative to remove industrial trans fats from the food supply.

Several scientific studies link the intake of trans-fats to depression and anxiety. For example, research shows that consuming trans fats can increase the risk of depression by as much as 48 percent.[32] Meanwhile, high intake of linoleic acid (the dominant omega-6 in seed oils) has been associated with greater odds of psychological distress and depression in adults.[33]

These unhealthy fats disrupt brain cell membranes, promote neuroinflammation, and interfere with neurotransmitter systems, essential for regulating mood and stress. They can alter serotonin, dopamine, and GABA signaling, resulting in brain fog, low motivation, anxiety, and depressive symptoms.

The effect is even worse when trans fats are combined with refined sugar, creating a dietary pattern that amplifies metabolic disruption, inflammatory cytokine release, and stress hormone imbalance—all pathways that increase anxiety and depressive states.[34] Cherie tells the story in *The Juice Lady's Guide to Juicing for Health* of how she completely turned her health around from chronic fatigue syndrome and fibromyalgia to vibrant health by eliminating all sugar, seed oils, refined and fast food, and eating only whole, organic foods and fresh vegetable juices. In three months, she felt like a new person and all the symptoms were gone.

How Industrial Seed Oils Can Contribute to Cancer, Specifically Breast and Colon

Cancer does not develop overnight. It arises over years through cumulative cellular damage, oxidative stress, chronic inflammation, and metabolic dysfunction. Industrial seed oils contribute to each of these processes in ways that are now well documented in biochemical and cancer research.

Because seed oils are highly polyunsaturated, their chemical structure is inherently unstable. During industrial processing—high-heat extraction, chemical solvents, and deodorization—and later during cooking and storage, they form oxidized lipid by-products. Once consumed, these damaged fats increase oxidative stress, injuring DNA, proteins, and cell membranes. Oxidative DNA damage is a recognized driver of cancer initiation.

Oxidized seed oils are also potent inflammatory triggers. Cancer thrives in inflammatory environments. When cell membranes are built from damaged fats, cellular signaling becomes impaired, apoptosis (programmed cell death) is disrupted, and immune surveillance weakens—core features of cancer biology. Seed oils further impair mitochondrial function, reducing the cell's ability to regulate energy production and eliminate damaged cells. Oxidized PUFAs increase free radical production and push cells toward inefficient energy metabolism, a hallmark of cancer cells.

Lipid peroxidation by-products—such as reactive aldehydes formed during seed oil oxidation—can bind directly to DNA and proteins, increasing the mutational burden. These compounds were never part of the human evolutionary diet, and chronic exposure overwhelms the body's detoxification capacity. Together, oxidative stress, inflammation, insulin resistance, and immune dysfunction create an internal environment that supports tumor development. While seed oils are not claimed to be the sole cause of cancer, evidence suggests they are significant contributors to the modern disease landscape.

Recent research strengthens this link. A 2025 study led by researchers at Weill Cornell Medicine and published in *Science* found that linoleic acid—the primary omega-6 fat in industrial seed oils—directly fueled the growth of aggressive cancer cells in laboratory models.[35]

The study focused on triple-negative breast cancer and showed that linoleic acid binds to the FABP5 protein in tumor cells, activating the mTORC1 growth pathway that drives cell metabolism and division. In mouse models, diets high in linoleic acid significantly increased tumor growth.[36]

Researchers also observed elevated linoleic acid and FABP5 levels in tumor tissue and blood samples from human patients, linking experimental findings to real-world cancer biology. While no single dietary factor causes cancer on its own, this study provides a clear mechanistic link between common seed oils and cancer progression.

Emerging evidence also implicates seed oils in colorectal cancer risk. Ultra-processed foods high in seed oils promote chronic inflammation in the colon, disrupting tissue repair and immune surveillance. Tumor samples from individuals with colon cancer show elevated levels of omega-6 fatty acids, which are common in soybean, canola, corn, safflower, and sunflower oils.[37]

Finally, seed oils negatively affect the gut microbiome. Short-chain fatty acids (SCFAs), particularly butyrate, are produced by beneficial gut bacteria and are essential for gut lining repair, controlling inflammation, regulating blood sugar, promoting healthy elimination, and maintaining immune balance. Seed oils disrupt beneficial bacteria and reduce butyrate production. Removing seed oils and replacing them with stable, traditional fats and oils helps reduce inflammation and restore microbial balance.

Cognitive Decline, Omega-3 Deficiency, and Alzheimer's and Dementia

Emerging research increasingly shows that the balance of dietary fats plays a critical role in brain health, particularly in neurodegenerative diseases such as Alzheimer's disease and dementia. Since modern Western diets are disproportionately high in omega-6 PUFAs, this imbalance has profound implications for neuronal structure, signaling, and inflammation control, all of which are crucial for maintaining cognitive function.

In *Genius Foods*, his bestselling book on brain health, Max Lugavere emphasizes that Western dietary patterns—especially pervasive consumption of processed seed oils—are linked to declines in cognitive resilience and an increased risk of both Alzheimer's disease and dementia. As he explains, DHA and EPA are essential to maintaining neuronal integrity, supporting synaptic function, and regulating inflammation. Low levels of these omega-3 fats correlate with cognitive impairment, and diets skewed toward omega-6 are associated with memory deficits, impaired learning, and accelerated neurodegeneration. Lugavere advocates for reducing inflammatory fats while prioritizing foods rich in omega-3s to support lifelong cognitive function and protect against dementia.

Animal studies reinforce these insights. In one PubMed-indexed study using an Alzheimer's disease mouse model, vegetable oils higher in alpha-linolenic acid (ALA, a plant omega-3) attenuated cognitive impairment relative to linoleic-rich oils, demonstrating a protective effect of omega-3s on memory, learning, and overall brain health.[38]

Human research mirrors these findings. Emerging studies have revealed sex-specific patterns in Alzheimer's and dementia patients, showing lower levels of unsaturated fatty acids, including omega-3s, in individuals with cognitive decline compared to healthy controls. These findings suggest that fatty acid imbalance is linked to neurodegenerative progression and may influence susceptibility to dementia and Alzheimer's disease.[39]

Taken together, the evidence paints a consistent picture: Dietary fat quality matters profoundly to brain health. Diets high in inflammatory seed oils and low in neuroprotective omega-3s shift the brain's biochemistry toward inflammation, oxidative stress, and impaired neuronal function, setting the stage for both Alzheimer's disease and dementia. Prioritizing foods rich in omega-3s—such as wild-caught fatty fish, algae, walnuts, chia, hempseeds, flax, and supplemental DHA—can help restore balance, protect neuronal integrity, and support long-term cognitive resilience.

Research suggests that populations in Greece, where the traditional Mediterranean diet is common, experience lower rates of dementia and Alzheimer's disease compared with many Western countries. Studies show that adherence to a diet rich in olive oil, vegetables, fish, and nuts is linked to slower cognitive decline, reduced neuroinflammation, and a lower overall risk of dementia. For example, the MICOIL pilot study in Greece found that extra-virgin olive oil high in polyphenols helped protect cognitive function in people with mild cognitive impairment, a condition that often precedes dementia.[40]

A large cohort study in the United States found that adults consuming at least 7 grams of olive oil per day (roughly half a tablespoon) had a 28 percent lower risk of dementia-related death compared with those who rarely consumed olive oil.[41] Furthermore, research on traditional Mediterranean populations shows that higher adherence to a Mediterranean diet is associated with a significantly reduced risk of dementia and cognitive decline in older adults.[42] While this doesn't mean that dementia is impossible in people who follow Mediterranean eating habits, it demonstrates the protective power of high-quality fats for the brain. For those looking to support cognitive health, it's not a bad idea to take a small shot of extra-virgin olive oil each day to help nourish the brain and potentially reduce risk over time.

How Seed Oils Affect the Skin: Acne, Psoriasis, and Eczema

Skin, hair, and nails are built from fats, along with proteins and minerals, and their health depends heavily on the quality and balance of fatty acids in the diet. Highly processed seed oils are rich in omega-6 linoleic acid, which, when consumed in excess, can promote systemic inflammation and oxidative stress—two key drivers of inflammatory skin conditions. Research shows that diets high in omega-6 fats relative to omega-3s are associated with increased inflammatory signaling in the skin, impairing its ability to repair, regenerate, and maintain a healthy barrier.[43]

One of the primary mechanisms involves lipid peroxidation. Polyunsaturated fats from seed oils are prone to oxidation, forming reactive by-products that can damage skin cells and disrupt normal keratinocyte function. Oxidative stress has been shown to play a direct role in the development and severity of acne, where oxidized lipids contribute to clogged pores, bacterial overgrowth, and increased inflammation.[44]

Inflammatory skin conditions such as eczema and psoriasis are also closely linked to immune dysregulation and fatty acid imbalance. Excess omega-6 intake can increase the production of inflammatory mediators derived from arachidonic acid; these mediators are elevated in both eczema and psoriasis lesions. Studies show that improving the ratio of omega-6s to omega-3s can help reduce inflammatory activity in the skin and support barrier repair.[45]

Chronic inflammation and oxidative stress also impairs collagen production, hair follicle function, and nail growth, contributing to dull skin, brittle nails, and increased hair shedding. The skin and hair follicles are particularly sensitive to inflammatory signaling and mitochondrial stress, which can disrupt growth cycles and slow regeneration.[46]

Seed Oils, Biofilms, and Parasitic Persistence

Biofilms are protective matrices formed by bacteria, fungi, and other microorganisms that allow them to adhere to tissues, evade immune defenses, and resist elimination. Chronic inflammation, oxidative stress, and excess damaged fats create an internal environment that supports biofilm formation—and diet plays a central role in shaping this terrain.

Highly processed seed oils are rich in omega-6 polyunsaturated fatty acids that oxidize easily, increasing inflammation and lipid peroxidation. Oxidized lipids have been shown to promote microbial survival strategies, including enhanced biofilm formation, by supplying inflammatory signals and structural components that microbes exploit.[47]

Inflamed, lipid-rich tissues provide an ideal substrate for biofilm adhesion, making pathogens harder for the immune system to detect and eliminate.[48] Parasites and pathogenic organisms also thrive in environments marked by impaired gut barrier function and inflammation driven by omega-6s that compromise mucosal immunity and favor persistence over clearance.[49]

Because biofilms are partially composed of lipids and fatty acid derivatives, excess oxidized fats may further stabilize these microbial communities. By contrast, dietary choices that reduce inflammatory fats and support bile flow and immune signaling have been shown to disrupt biofilm environments and improve microbial balance.[50]

Metabolic Issues Linked to Seed Oil Intake

Seed oils are not a neutral dietary choice. Their widespread use parallels the rise of modern metabolic disease, and research increasingly shows that these highly refined polyunsaturated fats disrupt normal physiology through multiple overlapping pathways.

Insulin Resistance and Glucose Dysregulation

One of the most significant metabolic effects of seed oil consumption is insulin resistance. Diets high in omega-6–rich fats—especially when combined with refined carbohydrates—impair cellular signaling, elevate blood sugar, and push the body toward type 2 diabetes. Animal studies show that omega-6 metabolites (oxylipins) correlate with increased insulin resistance under seed-oil–rich conditions.[51] Chronic insulin resistance promotes fat storage, metabolic slowdown, and systemic dysfunction.

Chronic Inflammation

Since seed oils are exceptionally high in linoleic acid (LA), they fuel pro-inflammatory signaling when consumed in excess relative to omega-3 fats. As mentioned previously, modern Western diets often exceed a 15:1 omega-6 to omega-3 ratio, far above ancestral levels. This imbalance drives persistent low-grade inflammation—a root contributor to metabolic disease—affecting blood vessels, adipose tissue, and insulin signaling.[52]

The National Library of Medicine notes that arachidonic acid, derived from omega-6 fats, significantly contributes to inflammatory cell membranes in Western diets.[53] As Dr. Dwight Lundell explains, without inflammation, cholesterol would not become trapped in blood vessel walls—making inflammation, not cholesterol, the primary driver of heart disease.[54]

Weight Gain, "Sick Fat," and Obesity

High intake of omega-6 seed oils is linked to increased adiposity and visceral fat accumulation. Animal studies show that seed-oil-based diets promote greater fat storage than diets using stable fats like coconut oil, independent of calorie intake.

Lipid peroxidation in fat tissue creates "adiposopathy" or "sick fat," where adipose cells secrete inflammatory cytokines instead of leptin, increasing risks of weight gain, heart disease, and metabolic dysfunction.[55] Obesity, in this context, is not a willpower issue but a metabolic disorder driven by inflammatory fats.

Fatty Liver, Lipids, and Gut Dysfunction

Seed oils contribute to nonalcoholic fatty liver disease by accumulating and oxidizing in liver tissue, impairing mitochondrial function and accelerating progression toward steatohepatitis.[56] They are also associated with dyslipidemia—high triglycerides, low HDL, and oxidized LDL—patterns strongly linked to cardiovascular disease.

Emerging evidence shows seed oils disrupt gut barrier integrity and microbiota balance, leading to metabolic endotoxemia and systemic inflammation.[57]

Hormonal Disruption and Appetite Dysregulation

Inflammatory lipid metabolites from seed oils disrupt adipokines such as leptin and adiponectin, impairing satiety signaling and promoting overeating.[58] Research shows linoleic acid suppresses fat oxidation, damages mitochondrial energy production, and promotes insulin resistance.[59]

Obesity rates rose alongside seed oil consumption—not traditional fats. Studies consistently show high-PUFA diets promote weight gain, while stable long-used fats support metabolic flexibility.[60]

A Web of Metabolic Disruption

Taken together, excessive seed oil consumption disrupts metabolism on multiple levels:

- Insulin resistance and glucose dysregulation
- Chronic inflammation
- Abnormal fat storage and obesity
- Fatty liver disease
- Dyslipidemia and cardiovascular risk
- Mitochondrial dysfunction
- Gut barrier breakdown
- Hormonal and appetite imbalance
- Increased cancer risk

These mechanisms reinforce one another, creating the metabolic storm underlying obesity, diabetes, cardiovascular disease, and declining population health.

Despite this, major institutions often promote seed oils as "heart-healthy." The global seed oil market is projected to reach $421 billion in 2026 and $598 billion by 2031. When evaluating nutrition science, funding sources and financial incentives matter. Human health is not complex by design. For thousands of years, people thrived on whole foods and traditional fats—long before industrial seed oils existed. When we replace foods created by nature with products engineered in labs, metabolic consequences should not surprise us.

Homicide and Aggression

One of the most controversial—and sobering—findings in nutritional neuroscience comes from a peer-reviewed longitudinal analysis of dietary fat intake across five Western countries —Argentina, Australia, Canada, the United Kingdom, and the United States—spanning 1961–2000. The researchers found that greater national availability of linoleic acid—the primary omega-6 fatty acid found in industrial seed oils such as soybean, corn, and canola oil—closely correlated with higher homicide mortality rates over time. The correlation coefficient was extraordinarily high ($r = 0.94$), meaning homicide rates rose almost in lockstep with increased linoleic acid consumption over several decades, and within each country, increased linoleic acid intake significantly predicted higher homicide mortality. While correlation does not prove causation, the authors discussed biologically plausible mechanisms involving neuroinflammation and disruption of neurotransmitter systems that regulate mood, impulse control, and aggression.[61]

Dr. Mark Hyman has spoken about this publicly and shared this disturbing research on his blog, highlighting seed oils as one of the modern dietary shifts linked to chronic inflammation and brain dysfunction, noting that over-consuming omega-6 fats like those in industrial seed oils can fuel inflammatory pathways and impair the balance with the brain, which is normally protected by omega-3s. This contributes to poor psychiatric outcomes, behavioral change, and broader health consequences.[62]

The Solution: Nurture the Brain with Healthy Fats

Your brain thrives on the fats it evolved on—not industrially refined seed oils, but whole, nourishing fats that support cellular repair, calm inflammation, and protect mitochondrial function. When oxidized oils are replaced with stable, traditional fats and carefully sourced plant oils, the brain is given the raw materials it needs to restore balance, resilience, and clarity. Extra-virgin olive oil, avocado oil, flaxseed oil, and black cumin seed oil provide protective compounds and fatty acids that work with the body rather than against it, helping rebalance omega intake and reduce inflammatory stress.

The next chapters provide everything you need to know about healthy fats and oils, showing how the right fats don't just fuel the body, but help restore it.

CHAPTER 3
Everything You Need to Know About Oils and Fats

Not All Seed Oils Are Created Equal

Welcome to your fats and oils handbook. If you've been confused about seed oils and fats—and what to choose for your recipes—this is your guide. We'll show you why you should select nut and fruit oils over industrial seed oils. We will show you what the healthiest seed oils are to buy. And we'll explain why animal fats, such as beef tallow and butter, are healthy options when properly sourced.

You'll learn why fats and oils behave differently in the body, how cooking temperature affects toxicity, why fat quality matters at the cellular level, and how choosing the healthiest fats and oils can help heal your body. In this chapter, you'll discover a whole new world regarding healthy fats and oils.

Beginning in the post–World War II era, the public was systematically confused about dietary fat. Fat was portrayed as dangerous, despite being an essential nutrient for human life. Our bodies don't merely tolerate fat—we are built on it. For most of human history, including during the Paleolithic era, natural fats fueled both the brain and the body long before modern dietary theories disrupted this understanding.

The human brain is made up of nearly 60 percent fat. Every nerve cell, every neurotransmitter, every electrical signal that allows you to think, feel, remember, focus, and stay calm depends on fat. Your nervous system is literally insulated by fat. It is responsible for focus, emotional regulation, hormone production, nervous system stability, and cell membrane integrity. Without adequate, quality fats, communication between the brain and body begins to break down. Fat is what allows the brain to stay resilient, flexible, and protected. It supports cognitive clarity. When we remove fat—or replace it with damaged, unstable fats—the brain pays the price.

It's important to understand the healthy fats vs the unhealthy fats. Not all fats are the same—and your body responds to each type of fat differently. Some fats are stable and nourishing (like saturated fats and monounsaturated fats), supporting the brain, hormones, and long-lasting energy. Others are fragile and easily damaged, especially polyunsaturated fats (omega-3 and omega-6). They must be kept in balance—because too much omega-6 and too little omega-3 can fuel inflammation and affect mood and brain function. The most harmful are trans fats, created through industrial processing and high heat; they disrupt cell membranes and promote oxidative stress.

Fat isn't the enemy. The wrong fats—and the lack of the right ones—are.

HEALTHY FATS VS. UNHEALTHY FATS

Healthy Oils

Almond oil
Animal fat including duck and lamb
Avocado oil
Beef tallow
Black seed oil (medicinal use)
Butter (grass-fed)
Coconut oil
Flaxseed oil
Ghee
Hemp seed oil
Macadamia nut oil
Olive oil
Pumpkin seed oil
Tigernut oil
Walnut oil

(Continued . . .)

Unhealthy Oils

- Canola oil (rapeseed oil)
- Corn oil
- Cottonseed oil
- Grapeseed oil
- Margarine
- Peanut oil
- Rice bran oil
- Safflower oil
- Shortening
- Soybean oil
- Sunflower oil
- Trans fats
- Vegetable oil

Fat has been misunderstood by modern generations. While we were taught to fear it, the body was quietly suffering from its absence—or worse, from the wrong kinds altogether. Fat is essential to human health, but only when it comes from stable, nourishing sources rather than damaged, toxic industrial ones.

The Four Types of Dietary Fats (and Why Structure Matters)

Dietary fats fall into four main categories based on their chemical structure. This structure determines how stable a fat is, how it behaves when heated, and how it affects inflammation, hormones, and cell membranes.

Saturated fats, as found in butter or coconut oil, contain no double bonds, making them the most stable fats. They are solid at room temperature and resist oxidation. Saturated fats are essential for cell membrane integrity, hormone production, and metabolic stability, and they are the safest fats for cooking.

Monounsaturated fats, like those in olive oil, contain one double bond. They are relatively stable, especially when gently heated, and are associated with improved metabolic health and reduced inflammation. Oleic acid, as found in olive oil, is the most well-known monounsaturated fat.

Polyunsaturated fats, which are prevalent in seed oils, contain two or more double bonds, making them fragile and highly prone to oxidation. While some polyunsaturated fats are essential in small amounts, they are easily damaged by heat, light, and industrial processing, forming inflammatory by-products.

Trans fats are industrially altered fats created through hydrogenation. They disrupt cell membranes, increase inflammation, and have no place in a health-supportive diet.

These categories form the foundation for understanding how fats function in the body and will be referenced throughout this chapter.

Fatty acids are the building blocks of all fats in the body, and their structure determines how fats affect digestion, energy, inflammation, and cellular health. Short-chain fatty acids, produced by beneficial gut bacteria, fuel the intestinal lining and support immune balance. Medium-chain fatty acids, found in coconut oil and dairy fat, are quickly converted into energy rather than stored. Long-chain fatty acids, present in animal fats, fish oil, nuts, and oils, form cell membranes, support hormone production, and provide essential fuel during metabolic stress—including protective fats around the heart. Very-long-chain fatty acids, found primarily in animal fats, play critical roles in skin integrity, nervous system insulation, vision, and reproduction. Because cell membranes are built from the fats we consume, relying on damaged industrial oils alters cellular signaling, metabolism, and long-term health.

Saturated and Unsaturated Fats: Setting the Record Straight

Saturated fats contain no double bonds, giving them a straight, tightly packed structure that makes them highly stable. This stability makes them resistant to oxidation and the safest fats for cooking.

Saturated fats were maligned for decades based on flawed assumptions rather than evidence. In reality, they are essential for cellular stability, hormone production, and metabolic health. They are the least likely fats to form toxic by-products when heated, and deficiencies can compromise cell membrane integrity.[1, 2, 3]

Were Tropical Oils Demonized to Steal the Market?

We now know coconut oil does not cause heart disease, so how was it labeled harmful? During World War II, disrupted trade routes from Southeast Asia created an opportunity for the domestic seed oil industry to dominate the market. At the same time, the 1950s ushered in widespread fear of saturated fat, driven by coordinated education and marketing campaigns.

As heart disease rose—despite being rare at the start of the twentieth century—cholesterol and saturated fat were blamed. This led to the lipid hypothesis, which claimed animal fats caused plaque buildup in arteries. Traditional foods like butter, eggs, and tallow were pushed aside, while vegetable oils were promoted as heart-healthy alternatives. Coconut oil, though cholesterol-free, was caught up in the backlash simply because it was saturated.

Today, research shows dietary cholesterol has little impact on blood cholesterol, and the lipid hypothesis has largely collapsed. Heart disease is now understood to be driven by inflammation, stress, smoking, poor diet, and metabolic dysfunction—not natural fats. In 2005, Cherie Calbom helped restore coconut oil's reputation with her book *The Coconut Diet*, contributing to its return as a kitchen staple and helping revive coconut farming communities worldwide.

The Truth About Polyunsaturated Fatty Acids (PUFAs) Revealed

Polyunsaturated fatty acids (PUFAs) are what comprise seed oils. They are volatile fatty acids because they have two or more double bonds that can be easily broken. For decades we were told PUFAs are good for us. A growing number of people who want to eat clean mistakenly believe that vegetable oils are a healthy choice. Often, these oils are used in packaged products and restaurant fare, but they are very susceptible to oxidation because of their polyunsaturated fatty acids. They also contribute to an imbalance in the omega-6-to-omega-3 fatty acid ratio. Add inflammation to the list of problems they cause, and you have serious issues regarding their consumption. This is related to the fact that polyunsaturated fats have unpaired electrons making them highly reactive.

Polyunsaturated fatty acids are good for us in their natural state, such as seeds, nuts, and salmon. We need them in small amounts. The problem arises when we eat too many of them and when we eat them in seed oils that are denatured and toxic, causing damage at the cellular level. They are the most vulnerable fatty acids when ultra-processed and subjected to high heat.

Why Have PUFAs Been So Revered?

For decades, PUFAs have been the "golden standard" of oils. Saturated fats (such as butter, beef and duck tallow, along with coconut oil) were demonized in the 1950s and for decades thereafter because they are saturated. PUFAs, which are unsaturated, were hailed as the heart-healthy alternatives. The American Heart Association and other health organizations have recommended replacing butter and other traditional cooking fats with margarine or vegetable oil. It was predicted that PUFAs might decrease LDL cholesterol. And here lies the twist: Correlation is not causation. Simply lowering a single biomarker doesn't necessarily translate into a good outcome. Recent research into PUFAs has cast a shadow on their once-sunny reputation and suggests that we've been looking at PUFAs all wrong.

PUFAs Compromise Cell Membranes

Eating vegetable oil can adversely affect the chemistry of cell membranes. When cell membrane integrity is compromised, we can experience the following:

- Drop in energy
- Nerves that don't fire efficiently
- Glands that malfunction
- Hormone levels drop
- Metabolism slows; we gain weight
- Cells become undernourished
- Weight loss is an uphill battle
- We feel tired; always hungry

PUFAs Surround Us

Everywhere we go, we are inundated with PUFAs—in our salad dressing, granola bars, and even in that so-called "healthy" restaurant meal cooked in canola oil. The typical American now gets 7 to 10 percent of their calories from PUFAs, while our ancestors likely consumed PUFAs at around 1 to 2 percent of their calories. The shift in food production and preparation, as well as the use of seed oils, has health implications that we're just now beginning to understand.

Take a look at your pantry. What oil is in your salad dressing? Even "healthy" snacks like gluten-free crackers, organic chips, and nut butters frequently contain PUFAs, such as canola, safflower, or sunflower oil, which are noted in fine print on hard-to-read labels. Eating out? The food on your plate was most likely sizzled in an oxidized, omega-6-rich seed oil with traces of hexane. The result of this dietary transition is a body that remains in a state of inflammatory and oxidative stress.

The Cholesterol Myth Exposed

We're discussing this topic because cholesterol is what set this controversy in motion nearly seventy years ago. Due to decades of intense media coverage, many people still believe fat and cholesterol are the primary causes of heart disease. Science has proven this is not true. The most important factor in heart disease prevention is reducing inflammation, as Cherie explains in *The Anti-Inflammation Diet*. The most accurate assessment involves inflammation markers such as histamine, C-reactive protein (CRP), erythrocyte sedimentation rate (ESR), and lipoprotein. Dr. Dwight Lundell, a heart surgeon, emphasizes that the focus should be on reducing inflammation and addressing root causes rather than simply lowering cholesterol with diet or medication.[4]

In reality, elevated cholesterol can reflect many underlying factors, including genetics, poor diet, lack of exercise, chronic stress, smoking, pregnancy, rapid weight loss, certain medications, unfiltered coffee, liver congestion, and other medical conditions. When cholesterol is high, it often signals deeper imbalances. A comprehensive approach should include dietary and lifestyle changes, exercise, stress reduction, gut and hormone evaluation, liver support, and inflammation reduction—rather than focusing solely on medication.

Is There Such a Thing as "High Cholesterol"?

According to Cate Shanahan, MD, the concept of "high cholesterol" as a disease is fundamentally flawed. Cholesterol is not a toxin or waste product—it is essential for life, forming cell membranes, hormones, and bile acids. As Dr. Shanahan explains in *Deep Nutrition* and *The Fatburn Fix*, "Cholesterol is not a poison. It is a vital substance that your body carefully regulates because you cannot live without it."

The body produces cholesterol on demand, especially during stress, inflammation, injury, or repair. When levels rise, cholesterol is often responding—not causing damage. Dr. Shanahan emphasizes that the real danger lies not in cholesterol itself, but in diets that promote oxidation of lipoproteins. Processed foods—and especially seed oils—are uniquely designed to promote oxidation, making cholesterol-carrying particles fragile and prone to damage.

"Cholesterol-containing LDL only becomes dangerous when it is damaged (oxidized). And what damages it most is seed oil."[5]

Scientific evidence supports this distinction: Oxidized LDL—not total LDL—is strongly associated with atherosclerosis and cardiovascular risk. Cholesterol particles become harmful primarily when exposed to oxidative stress, inflammation, and unstable polyunsaturated fats.[6]

Dr. Shanahan also challenges the assumption that lowering cholesterol improves outcomes. Large scientific reviews show cholesterol levels alone are poor predictors of heart disease, particularly in metabolically healthy individuals and older adults. Some studies even associate higher cholesterol with greater longevity,

Rather than fixating on cholesterol numbers, Dr. Shanahan urges attention to fat quality, mitochondrial health, and inflammation. Traditional diets rich in stable fats and natural cholesterol supported cardiovascular health long before industrial seed oils entered the food supply. As she summarizes: "Heart disease is not a cholesterol problem. It's a problem of damaged fats, damaged metabolism, and damaged mitochondria."

In this context, cholesterol is not the enemy—it is a biological repair molecule, repeatedly blamed for damage caused by inflammatory diets, oxidative stress, and ultra-processed oils.

CHOLESTEROL—MYTH VS. REALITY

Myth:
High cholesterol causes heart disease.

Reality:
Cholesterol is a vital, protective substance that the body produces for cell membranes, hormones, bile acids, and tissue repair. According to Dr. Cate Shanahan, cholesterol itself is not harmful—it becomes problematic only when it is damaged or oxidized, most often due to systemic antioxidant depletion and unstable fats from industrial seed oils. She says, "Cholesterol is not a poison. It's a repair molecule. The problem isn't cholesterol—it's what damages it."

Myth:
Cholesterol should be treated as the enemy.

Reality:
Cholesterol is best understood as a nutrient, not a toxin. Elevated HDL cholesterol often signals healthy eating patterns and a body that's better equipped to manage stress, support immunity, and maintain reproductive health. Dr. Cate warns that chasing cholesterol numbers too low is potentially dangerous.

How We Got Fooled—History, the Lipid Hypothesis, and the War on Tropical Oils

We now know that coconut oil does not cause heart disease and, in fact, supports heart health and metabolic function. So how did it become demonized? As we mentioned earlier, during World War II, shipping routes from Southeast Asia were disrupted, limiting access to tropical oils and allowing the seed oil industry to dominate the market. In the 1950s, public opinion began turning against saturated fats through coordinated educational and marketing campaigns. This shift coincided with a sharp rise in heart disease, which had been rare at the start of the twentieth century but became the leading cause of death in the US by the 1950s.[7, 8]

Researchers searched urgently for a cause, yet few examined changes in the American diet. Instead, a new explanation emerged, and cholesterol was blamed. Because cholesterol was found primarily in animal foods—meat, eggs, butter, and cheese—these foods were labeled dangerous. This led to the "lipid hypothesis," which claimed saturated fat and cholesterol caused arterial plaque. (It was not a cause, but a response to irritated, inflamed arteries.) Traditional fats were pushed out, and vegetable oils were promoted as heart-healthy replacements. Although tropical oils contain no cholesterol, they were targeted simply because they are saturated. Modern research has since shown that dietary cholesterol has little to no effect on blood cholesterol levels.[9]

Many researchers now reject the lipid hypothesis as the root cause of heart disease altogether, recognizing the roles of inflammation, smoking, stress, obesity, poor diet, and metabolic dysfunction instead.

After World War II, seed oil consumption increased dramatically. Mary Enig documented that while butter intake declined, hydrogenated vegetable oils, margarine, and shortening surged. By 1950, vegetable oil consumption had more than tripled. Enig's work—*The Oiling of America and Coconut: In Support of Good Health in the 21st Century*—details how these shifts were accompanied by aggressive campaigns against saturated fats.[10]

In *The Coconut Diet*, Cherie Calbom explains how coconut oil—once widely consumed and promoted as healthy in the 1930s—was suddenly vilified. In 1986, the American Soybean Association distributed the "Fat Fighter Kit" to oppose tropical oil imports.[11] The Center for Science in the Public Interest followed with its 1988 booklet *Saturated Fat Attack*, which Dr. Enig later criticized for serious biochemical errors.[12]

Media attacks escalated. In 1988, Phil Sokolof placed newspaper ads depicting coconut oil as a "health bomb," accusing companies of "poisoning America."[13]

Tropical oil producers—primarily in the Philippines, Malaysia, and Indonesia—lacked the resources to counter these narratives. Yet experts testified otherwise. Dr. George Blackburn of Harvard reported that coconut oil has a neutral effect on blood cholesterol, even when it is the sole fat source (Calbom, *The Coconut Diet*). Mary Enig noted that tropical oils have been consumed safely for thousands of years, and former Surgeon General Dr. C. Everett Koop dismissed the scare as "foolishness."[14]

Finally, physiology tells its own story. The heart relies heavily on saturated fats—specifically palmitic (C16) and stearic (C18) acids—during metabolic stress. Research confirms that long-chain fatty acids are essential fuels for the heart, especially during fasting or stress. Coconut oil, along with butter and other traditional fats, provides these critical fatty acids.

Seed Oils Not Recommended for Use

Not all oils belong in a healthy kitchen. Many modern seed oils are highly processed, unstable, and prone to oxidation, especially when exposed to heat, light, and oxygen. These oils are typically extracted with chemical solvents, such as hexane, and then refined, bleached, and deodorized at extremely high temperatures. The result is an oil far removed from its original source, which can contribute to inflammation, oxidative stress, and metabolic dysfunction. These oils are often referred to as the "Hateful 8," and we expand that list in this chapter to include additional oils that should also be avoided or used with extreme caution.

Oils to Avoid

Oils to avoid in cooking and in packaged foods such as crackers, chips, condiments, and frozen meals include soybean oil, canola oil, cottonseed oil, grapeseed oil, sunflower oil, safflower oil, rice bran oil, peanut oil, and palm oil (depending on the source). Read ingredient labels carefully.

These oils are typically high in linoleic acid, a fragile omega-6 polyunsaturated fat that oxidizes easily. When consumed in excess—as is common in modern diets—these oils can drive chronic inflammation and increase lipid oxidation.

Palm oil deserves special mention. While traditionally produced palm oil can be stable, most palm oil used in processed foods is highly refined and poorly sourced, raising both health and environmental concerns. For this reason, palm oil should be avoided unless the source and processing are clearly known and trusted.

CLEVERLY DISGUISED NAMES FOR SEED OIL

- Vegetable oil
- Vegetable oil blend
- Interesterified oil
- Modified vegetable oil
- Fractionated oil
- Oleic sunflower oil/high oleic oil (still seed oil)
- Soy lecithin
- Sunflower lecithin
- Rapeseed lecithin
- Egg lecithin
- Mono- and diglycerides
- DATEM (diacetyl tartaric acid ester of mono- and diglycerides) — commonly sourced from vegetable oils, particularly soybean oil and palm oil.
- Polysorbates (e.g., polysorbate 80)
- Glycerin / glycerol esters of fatty acids
- Propylene glycol esters of fatty acids
- Sorbitan monostearate
- Stearates
- Hydrogenated, partially hydrogenated, fully hydrogenated
- SSL(Sodium stearoyl-2-lactylate)
- Calcium stearoyl
- Sucrose esters
- Tocopherols (Vitamin E) — frequently used as preservatives and often derived from soybean or other vegetable oils.

Lipid Oxidation, Storage, and Rancidity

Fats degrade when exposed to heat, light, air, and time. Even healthy oils can become harmful if stored improperly. Oxidized and rancid oils contribute to oxidative stress and inflammation.

Practical guidelines:

- Store oils in dark glass containers
- Keep oils away from heat and light
- Refrigerate delicate oils such as flaxseed oil and nut oils
- Discard oils that smell bitter, stale, or "paint-like"

This is one reason industrial seed oils are so problematic—they are often oxidized long before they reach your kitchen.

Cold-Pressed, Expeller-Pressed, and Solvent-Extracted Oils

- Cold-pressed oils are extracted mechanically below 122°F, preserving nutrients and flavor.
- Expeller-pressed oils use mechanical pressure at 140°F to 210°F without chemicals.
- Solvent-extracted oils use hexane or other chemical solvents and extreme heat, often over 500°F, degrading fats and producing toxic by-products.

Fat-Soluble Vitamins: Why Fat Is a Delivery System

Fats are essential for the absorption of vitamins A, D, E, and K. Low-fat diets impair the absorption of these nutrients, affecting immunity, hormones, bone health, vision, and brain function. Traditional fats such as butter, ghee, and tallow provide these vitamins in highly bioavailable forms.

Which Fats Are Essential and Which Are Not

It is recommended that 20 to 35 percent of calories come from fat. Essential fats are those the body cannot synthesize—omega-3 and omega-6 fats.

Modern diets contain excessive omega-6 fatty acids and insufficient omega-3 fatty acids, leading to chronic inflammation. Western diets often reach omega-6: omega-3 ratios of 15–17:1, while the ideal ratio is closer to 1:1–4:1.[15]

Trans Fats: A Dangerous Industrial Creation

Trans fats—also called trans fatty acids—are a type of unsaturated fat in which the hydrogen atoms around a carbon–carbon double bond are arranged in a trans configuration rather than the usual cis form found in nature. They are created during the manufacturing of seed oils that are hydrogenated, such as shortening and margarine. Manufacturers take liquid seed oil and add hydrogen to make it more solid and shelf-stable. This causes unsaturated fat molecules to flip into the trans configuration rather than fully saturate. They have often been labeled as "partially hydrogenated vegetable oils." They raise LDL and lower HDL, increasing the risk of heart disease. Many countries have banned them for this reason. Why are we still allowing them in manufactured food? People don't even know they are there.[16]

These products contain the most trans fat:

- Margarine, spreads, and shortening
- Packaged and processed foods
- Ramen noodles, soup cups
- Microwave popcorn
- Fast food—fries, fried chicken, fried fish, and anything else deep-fried
- Frozen foods—frozen pies, pot pies, waffles, pizza, breaded fish sticks
- Commercial baked goods—doughnuts, cookies, and cakes
- Snack foods like chips and crackers
- Boxed breakfast cereals
- Candy
- Toppings and dips—nondairy creamers, whipped toppings, bean dip, gravy mixes, and salad dressings

A Note on Smoke Points, Tradition, and Real Life

Have you ever left oil in a pan with the heat on, only to turn around for a minute and return to find it smoking? Every fat and oil has a smoke point. This point indicates the temperature at which the oil or fat begins to break down and smoke. When this happens, the oil releases free radicals and other harmful compounds.

Typically, polyunsaturated fats have a low smoke point, which means they oxidize easily and form toxic by-products when heated. Fruit and nut oils have higher smoke points, making them more durable during cooking. Most animal fats have the highest smoke points and the greatest stability, which is why they have been used for centuries for cooking.

Dr. Cate Shanahan makes an important point about smoke points and real-world cooking. For generations, Italians cooked everything with olive oil—including frying—without obsessing over exact temperatures. They trusted olive oil because it was fresh, locally produced, and tasted good. Lower-quality, non-virgin oils, on the other hand, were historically used for fueling lamps and machinery, not for nourishing the body. The issue is not that olive oil instantly becomes toxic at a certain temperature, but that modern industrial seed oils contain polyunsaturated fatty acids that are oxidized and degraded (often into potent toxins) before they ever reach the pan. Fresh, properly produced olive oil (not cut with other oils) contains antioxidants that help protect it from oxidation during cooking, whereas refined seed oils oxidize easily and break down into harmful by-products.

Smoke Point Categories

- Low smoke point: 300°F–350°F
  These oils are suitable for low-heat cooking, light sautéing, salad dressings, and drizzling. Butter has a smoke point between 302°F and 350°F (choose only pastured, grass-fed).
- Medium smoke point: 350°F–375°F
  Suitable for sautéing, baking, and stir-frying. Olive oil and coconut oil are good choices for medium-heat cooking, along with avocado, almond, and macadamia nut oils.

- High smoke point: 375°F or higher
  Ideal for frying, searing, and grilling. Avocado, almond, and macadamia nut oils are good for high-heat cooking. Beef tallow has a smoke point of 480°F, and ghee has a smoke point of 485°F (choose only pastured, grass-fed).

FRUIT AND NUT OIL SMOKE POINTS

- Olive oil: 350°F–410°F
- Coconut oil: 350°F
- Avocado oil: 480°F–520°F
- Macadamia nut oil: 410°F
- Almond oil: 420°F
- Sesame oil: 350°F–425°F

ANIMAL FAT SMOKE POINTS

- Butter: 302°F–350°F
- Beef tallow: 480°F
- Ghee: 485°F

Benefits of Individual Oils and Fats

Olive Oil

Olive oil is a monounsaturated fat rich in oleic acid (71 percent), which has been shown to reduce inflammation and positively influence genes linked to cancer.[17] Large population studies associate olive oil consumption with reduced risk of heart disease and stroke, including a 2004 analysis of 841,000 participants. Olive oil contains apolipoprotein A-IV (ApoA-IV), which helps prevent platelet aggregation—a key factor in heart attacks and strokes.[18] A 2022 Harvard study found that consuming just ½ tablespoon daily was associated with a 19 percent lower risk of mortality.[19]

Extra-virgin olive oil also supports gut health and is one of the richest dietary sources of squalene, a compound linked to reduced cancer risk.[20] Diets rich in monounsaturated fats like olive oil improve insulin sensitivity and reduce inflammation.[21]

Coconut Oil

Virgin coconut oil has demonstrated anti-stress and antioxidant effects in animal models, including lower cortisol, cholesterol, triglycerides, glucose, and improved brain antioxidant status. Published in the journal *Experimental and Therapeutic Medicine* and believed to be the first study of its kind, researchers evaluated the anti-stress and antioxidant effects of virgin coconut oil in mice with stress-induced injuries. Researchers concluded it functions as an "anti-stress functional oil."[22] Coconut oil qualifies as a functional food—defined as providing health benefits beyond basic nutrition.[23]

In humans, a four-month study combining coconut oil with green tea polyphenols significantly reduced anxiety in patients with multiple sclerosis.[24]

Avocado Oil

Avocado oil is rich in oleic acid, omega-9 fats, carotenoids, and antioxidants that support cardiovascular, skin, and eye health. Animal studies show it reduces blood pressure similarly to losartan and lowers triglycerides and LDL cholesterol without reducing HDL.[25]

Macadamia Nut Oil

High in oleic acid, macadamia oil has been shown to reduce oxidative stress, lower LDL cholesterol, support gut health, and reduce heart-disease risk.[26, 27]

Almond Oil

Almond oil supports cholesterol transport, raises HDL, lowers LDL, and provides vitamin E, which is associated with reduced cognitive decline and macular degeneration.[28] It may also help regulate blood sugar.

Black Seed Oil

Black seed oil (*Nigella sativa*) is widely studied for anti-inflammatory, antioxidant, anticancer, and antiparasitic effects driven by thymoquinone. Research shows it induces apoptosis in cancer cells while sparing healthy cells and inhibits tumor growth and angigenesis.[29]

It also demonstrates antiparasitic activity[30] and supports the immune system, blood sugar balance, liver protection, and oxidative stress reduction.

Flaxseed and Hempseed Oils

Flaxseed oil is rich in omega-3 ALA, supporting heart health, reducing inflammation, supporting digestion, and supporting mental health. Hempseed oil provides omega-3s, GLA, and arginine, supporting cardiovascular function, inflammation control, circulation, and mood.

MCT Oil

MCT oil delivers caprylic (C8) and capric (C10) acids that are rapidly converted to energy rather than stored as fat. Studies show increased fat oxidation, energy expenditure, and ketone production—beneficial for metabolic and cognitive health.[31] CTs also exhibit antimicrobial properties and are often better tolerated in compromised digestion.[32]

Pumpkin Seed Oil

Pumpkin seed oil supports heart health, hair growth, prostate health, urinary function, and parasite resistance.[33]

Sesame Seed Oil

Sesame oil lowers blood pressure, improves blood sugar control, reduces inflammation, and may help arthritis.[34]

Walnut Oil

Walnut oil supports heart and brain health and improves lipid profiles due to its omega-3 content.

Animal Fats: Tallow, Butter, and Ghee

Beef tallow contains stearic acid (≈22 percent) and oleic acid (≈39 percent). Stearic acid stimulates metabolism, while oleic acid supports mitochondrial function, glucose balance, and satiety. Tallow provides fat-soluble vitamins A, D, E, K, and CLA, which may help prevent atherosclerosis and support weight management.[35] Grass-fed butter supplies vitamins A and D and CLA linked to metabolic and anticancer benefits.[36]

Ghee, a clarified butter, is rich in butyric acid, which supports gut healing and immune function and may benefit inflammatory bowel conditions.[37]

Individual Fat Tolerance

Fat tolerance varies based on bile flow, liver and gallbladder function, and gut health. Digestive symptoms during transition often indicate a need for gradual introduction and digestive support—not fat intolerance. Supporting liver health, chewing well, easing fat intake, and using probiotics can improve tolerance.

Replacing industrial seed oils with properly sourced fats restores omega balance, reduces oxidative stress, and supports metabolic, hormonal, and cellular health. The fats you choose shape your inflammation levels, energy, and long-term vitality.

CHAPTER 4

Nourishing Recipes with Nature's Healthiest Fats and Oils

In this chapter, we highlight the life-giving qualities of healthy fats and oils that add texture and flavor to your cooking and support your overall health. From the classic savory taste of olive oil, the tropical creaminess of coconut oil, the buttery smoothness of macadamia nut oil, and the vivid freshness of avocado oil, to the delicate nutty taste of almond oil, each offers its own character. Grass-fed pasture butter gives dishes richness and creaminess to food and flakiness to pie crusts. Beef tallow adds a velvety texture and meaty flavor. Ghee introduces a rich buttery taste. These recipes bring out natural flavors, demonstrating how the right oils and fats can turn our daily meals into rich sources of nutrition.

We hope you enjoy these recipes for a lifetime! By choosing healthier fats and oils in place of highly processed seed oils, you support a more balanced intake of omega-3 to omega-6 fatty acids. This shift can help calm inflammation and reduce oxidative stress—two factors closely linked to overall metabolic health. Over time, improving the quality of the fats you eat can contribute to better weight regulation and support cardiovascular, metabolic, gut, nervous system and immune function. Simply put, selecting high-quality oils and fats is a powerful way to invest in your long-term health and vitality. Heal yourself one meal at a time.

Tips for Healthy Cooking

1. Eat real foods and choose organic produce as much as possible to avoid pesticides.
2. Select whole organic grains whenever possible to avoid glyphosate contamination and GMOs
3. Avoid foods with soy.
4. Choose sea salt instead of refined table salt.
5. Select low-glycemic, natural sweeteners such as stevia and monk fruit whenever possible. When called for, choose organic pure maple syrup, coconut nectar, or honey.
6. Avoid foods with additives, preservatives, and dyes.
7. Make sure to use good-quality cookware like American stainless surgical steel; that is the highest quality you can get. If you cook with Teflon or other nonstick cookware, it will leach toxins into your food.
8. If you are using an air fryer, make sure it is high-quality stainless steel (ideally American-made stainless steel) so that no toxins leach into your food.

We hope you enjoy the nourishing recipes in the pages that follow, which contain a variety of healthy, flavorful fats and oils.

RECIPES WITH OLIVE OIL

Ways to Use Olive Oil

With a fruity flavor and a hint of bitterness and pungency, olive oil has been used for centuries to prepare food and promote healing. Depending on harvesting and processing, flavors can vary widely across different varieties. Olives from early harvesting tend to be more bitter and pungent, whereas late harvests are typically fruitier. Olive oil is used in various ways in food preparation, including salad dressing, mayonnaise, marinades, sautéing, frying, grilling, baking, and drizzling. Due to its higher smoke point, it is highly versatile in the kitchen.

Make Your Own Homemade Salad Dressing

Why buy store-bought salad dressings? Almost all of them are made with unhealthy seed oils and sugars. They do not support health. Additionally, they are a waste of money when you can make your own that tastes even better, using ingredients that are actually good for you, and keep it in a jar in the fridge where it will last for months.

LIANA'S BASIC SALAD DRESSING OR VINAIGRETTE

The basic premise of a salad dressing is to combine oil with an acid, such as lemon juice or vinegar. If you have these ingredients on hand, you can make your own dressing for tastier, more exciting salads. Then you can add other ingredients for a variety of flavors.

Total time: 5 minutes
Makes ⅓ cup

Ingredients:

⅓ cup extra-virgin olive oil, coconut oil, MCT, or avocado oil
2 tablespoons apple cider vinegar or balsamic vinegar (make sure the balsamic doesn't contain sugar or sulfites)
1 tablespoon fresh lemon juice
Sea salt and pepper, to taste

Instructions:

1. Add all the ingredients to a bowl and whisk until well combined. Season with sea salt and pepper, if desired.
2. Refrigerate in an airtight container or jar. This basic salad dressing lasts for up to two months.

Tip: Coconut oil is solid at temperatures below 76°F. Care must be taken when incorporating the oil at lower temperatures, and it's best eaten immediately rather than stored in the fridge.

Variations:

- Caesar Salad Dressing: Add ¼ teaspoon mustard powder, 2 tablespoons nutritional yeast, ½ teaspoon honey, 1 teaspoon minced garlic, ¼ teaspoon salt, and ¼ teaspoon pepper.
- Cheesy Dressing: Add 1 tablespoon nutritional yeast and ½ teaspoon sea salt.
- Citrus Salad Dressing: Add the juice of 1 orange and 1 grapefruit.
- Creamy Avocado Dressing: Add 1 seeded and peeled avocado and either mash it or blend it into the dressing.
- Garlic Salad Dressing: Add 2 teaspoons minced garlic or 1 teaspoon garlic powder.
- Ginger Salad Dressing: Add 1-inch piece of ginger, minced.
- Honey Mustard Dressing: Add 2 tablespoons honey, 1 tablespoon mustard powder, 1 teaspoon minced garlic, ¼ teaspoon sea salt, and ¼ teaspoon black pepper.
- Hummus Salad Dressing: Add 2 tablespoons hummus.
- Lime Vinaigrette: Use lime instead of lemon and add a bit of honey, if you want to make your dressing sweet.
- Mango Salad Dressing: Add 1 peeled and seeded mango and either mash it or blend it into the dressing.
- Mustard Vinaigrette: Add 1 teaspoon minced garlic, 1 tablespoon mustard, ¼ teaspoon black pepper, and ¼ teaspoon salt.
- Roasted Sunflower Seed Dressing: Add 2 tablespoons organic SunButter and mix until smooth and creamy.

- Sesame Ginger Dressing: Add 1 tablespoon toasted sesame seeds, 1 tablespoon grated ginger, 1 tablespoon organic SunButter, and 1 tablespoon tahini, and mix until smooth.
- Spicy Salad Dressing: Add ⅛ teaspoon cayenne pepper.
- Sweet Salad Dressing: Add 1 tablespoon honey.
- Tahini Salad Dressing: Add 2 tablespoons tahini.
- Thai Curry Dressing: Add 2 tablespoons green or red curry paste.
- Turmeric Salad Dressing: Add 1 teaspoon turmeric powder for extra health benefits.

PLANT-BASED TACO SALAD

Liana's recipe contains healthy omega-3 fats from olive oil, walnuts, and avocado.

Total time: 10 minutes
Serves 4

Ingredients:

Vegan Taco Mix

1½ cups walnuts
1 cup sun-dried tomatoes
2 tablespoons extra-virgin olive oil
1 teaspoon sage
1 teaspoon cumin
1 teaspoon fennel seeds
1 teaspoon thyme
1 teaspoon rosemary
1 teaspoon oregano
Pinch of black pepper
Pinch of cayenne pepper
¼ teaspoon Redmond Real Salt Taco Seasoning

Salad:

8 cups mixed greens, including kale, spinach, and lettuce
1 cup broccoli sprouts
1 avocado, sliced
1 tablespoon nutritional yeast
Sliced avocado to top salads, optional

Dressing:

2 tablespoons extra-virgin olive oil
1 lemon, juiced
Dash of sea salt
Dash of pepper

Instructions:

1. Place all the ingredients for the taco mix in a blender and blend until well combined.
2. Divide the salad greens and broccoli sprouts between four bowls.
3. Sprinkle the taco mix over each salad.
4. Top each salad with avocado slices.
5. Mix the salad dressing in a bowl and then pour it over the salad.
6. Finish by sprinkling nutritional yeast on top of each salad, and add sliced avocado, if desired.

GRASS-FED BEEF BURRITOS/TACOS

A classic staple eaten once per week in Liana's household. This recipe contains healthy fats from grass-fed beef, avocado, and olive oil. You can make this recipe into a burrito or a taco, depending on whether you wrap it or put it in a shell! Choose an organic soft tortilla for a burrito, and a non-GMO corn taco shell for a taco. Either way, the result can be a delicious feast for just you alone or for an entire family. The spices are all super for the brain and delicious. You can even use lettuce wraps for burritos if you want to reduce carbs. And you can choose a different meat, too! Chicken and fish also make great burrito and taco fillers. For a vegan option, you can use beans instead of beef.

Total time: 25 minutes
Serves 4

Ingredients:

2 tablespoons extra-virgin olive oil
1 teaspoon turmeric powder, divided
¼ teaspoon black pepper
1 pound ground organic grass-fed and grass-finished ground beef
1 small yellow onion, chopped
2 large garlic cloves, diced
1½ teaspoons ground cumin
½ teaspoon paprika
¼ teaspoon Redmond Real Salt
¼ teaspoon pepper
1 teaspoon chili powder or ¼ teaspoon cayenne pepper, optional (if you want it a little spicy)
4 tortillas, 4 lettuce wraps, or 8 taco shells

Fillings (your choice):

¾ cup organic sour cream or vegan sour cream
1 cup nutritional yeast
½ cup grated carrot
1 cup diced lettuce
1 avocado, cubed
1 pepper, diced
Fresh chopped cilantro
1 handful of broccoli sprouts
Ground beef (about 5 oz per person) or 16 ounces black beans (soaked, cooked, soft) or

Instructions:

1. Heat the oil in a large frying pan over medium heat. Add ½ teaspoon turmeric and black pepper. Sauté for 1 minute or until sizzling. Add

the beef and cook for 3 to 4 minutes, stirring frequently, until it turns brown.

2. Add the onion, garlic, cumin, ½ teaspoon turmeric, paprika, salt, pepper, and chili powder, if using, to the meat and stir. Cook for 7 minutes, or until the vegetables are tender and the flavors have combined well.
3. Place ¼ cup of meat into each tortilla, or 2 tablespoons into a taco shell, and then add your fillings of choice.

CAULIFLOWER POPCORN

A delicious take on healthy popcorn, made with a twist with cauliflower. Also goes great with broccoli. Recipe by Liana.

Total time: 10 minutes
Serves 4

Ingredients:

2½ tablespoons extra-virgin olive oil or coconut oil
½ cup nutritional yeast
¾ teaspoon sea salt
1 head cauliflower, chopped into bite-sized pieces

Instructions:

1. Preheat oven to 325°F.
2. In a large bowl, mix the oil, nutritional yeast, and salt until combined. Add the cauliflower pieces to the bowl and toss until the pieces are well coated.
3. Add to a baking tray and bake for 20 minutes until just golden brown.

Tip: Add 1 tablespoon sesame seeds for extra flavor.

GREEN SPROUT SALAD

The ultimate green salad made from dark leafy greens, one of the most powerful things for reducing stress and anxiety, all together in one bowl! This salad is quite surprising as it is built on a foundation of herbs, and it is so simple yet really flavorful and refreshing. It is also ridiculously high in antioxidants and magnesium, so you will feel better immediately—I promise! Try this salad. It is also quite filling. Recipe by Liana.

Total time: 15 minutes
Serves 1

Ingredients:

1 avocado, cubed
1 cup fresh parsley leaves
1 small cucumber, sliced
1 cup fresh cilantro leaves
1 cup broccoli sprouts
1½ cups grated broccoli
1 lemon
1 tablespoon olive oil
Sea salt and pepper, to taste

Instructions:

1. Add all the ingredients in a bowl except for the lemon, olive oil, sea salt, and pepper. Toss until well combined.
2. Squeeze lemon juice over the salad and drizzle the olive oil. Season with salt and pepper, to taste.

GUACAMOLE GREENS CHICKEN SALAD

This is my (Liana's) favorite salad as of late; I call this the party salad. It makes me feel like I'm on the beach, or at a party somewhere that I love with people that I enjoy. This is also my go-to salad when I do long days at Complete Wellness, the medical health center where I work in New York

City seeing patients. This salad makes me excited for lunch and helps me to stay energized until dinner. It has some Mexican flavors with a lime vinaigrette and corn chips, and some satisfying protein from delightfully juicy baked chicken breast.

Total time: 25 minutes
Serves 1

Ingredients:

1 organic chicken breast
½ head small lettuce, diced
¼ cup cherry tomatoes, chopped in half
½ cucumber, sliced and cut into slices and then halves
½ carrot, grated
1 tablespoon fresh cilantro
½ avocado, mashed
1 tablespoon purple onion, cut into small pieces
2 tablespoons extra-virgin olive oil
1 lime, juiced
Sea salt to taste
Pepper to taste
½ cup organic corn chips or cassava chips

Instructions:

1. Preheat the oven to 450°F. Place the chicken breast on a baking tray and bake for 15 to 20 minutes until cooked through.
2. While the chicken cooks, make the salad by adding the lettuce, tomatoes, cucumber, carrot, onion, and cilantro into the bowl. Add the avocado and toss well.
3. In a separate bowl, whisk together the olive oil, lime, salt, and pepper and then pour over salad.
4. Slice the chicken or cut into cubes and then add to the salad, add the corn chips, toss well, and enjoy!

Tip: Bake chicken for a shorter time at a higher temperature for the juiciest chicken ever. Baking for 15 to 20 minutes at 450°F will give you the juiciest chicken breast you have ever eaten. Baking chicken at 30 minutes at 350°F or lower will make for dry meat.

SUPERFOOD KALE SALAD

Total time: 10 minutes
Serves 3

Ingredients:

- 1 bunch of kale, center ribs and stems removed (save the stems and ribs for juicing or eating later)
- 1 avocado
- 1 tablespoon apple cider vinegar
- 1 tablespoon flaxseed oil
- ½ tablespoon pumpkin seed oil
- ¾ teaspoon sea salt or 2 teaspoons Liquid Aminos
- 4 tablespoons nutritional yeast
- 2 tablespoons sunflower seeds
- 2 tablespoons pumpkin seeds

Instructions:

1. Tear the kale leaves into small pieces and place in a large bowl.
2. Massage the avocado into the pieces of kale with your fingers, covering the kale with avocado.
3. Add the remaining ingredients to the bowl and stir, or continue to massage the mixture with your fingers, until everything is well combined.

Tip: Add 2 teaspoons garlic powder for extra immune-boosting benefits.

CHERIE'S GINGER LIME DRESSING

Total time: 5 minutes
Makes 4 servings

Ingredients:

¼ cup fresh lime juice
¼ cup extra-virgin olive oil or avocado oil
¼ cup purified water
2 tablespoons tamari or coconut aminos
2 tablespoons fresh mint
1 tablespoon fresh cilantro
1 teaspoon ginger root powder or 2 teaspoons grated ginger
1 thin slice red chili pepper, chopped, or a dash of cayenne pepper
2 teaspoons of raw honey or coconut nectar
1 teaspoon sea salt

Instruction:

Mix all ingredients in a blender.

CHERIE'S SIMPLE OLIVE OIL MAYONNAISE

You can make your own mayonnaise that's free of sugar, unhealthy seed oils, and preservatives.

Total time: 10 minutes
Makes 1 cup

Ingredients:

1 raw free-range or pastured egg
1 teaspoon Dijon mustard
1 teaspoon fresh lemon juice
1 cup extra-virgin olive oil (or a combination of ½ olive oil and ½ avocado oil).

Instructions:

1. It is very important to start with all ingredients at room temperature.
2. Using a blender or food processor, combine the raw egg, mustard, and lemon juice.
3. Blend and add the oil in a thin but steady stream until the mixture is quite thick. If the mixture won't thicken, add more oil.

Variation: you could add a handful of fresh herbs at the start, which will give the mayonnaise a delightful color and a different flavor. Also, to provide the mayonnaise more "zing," you may add a small anchovy fillet or a few capers.

CHERIE'S MINT MARINADE

Total time: 10 minutes
Serves 4

Ingredients:

¼ cup tamari or coconut aminos
1 tablespoon raspberry vinegar
1 tablespoon avocado oil or olive oil
1 tablespoon chopped fresh mint or 1 teaspoon dried
1 teaspoon monk fruit sweetener
¼ teaspoon freshly ground black pepper

Instruction:

Whisk together all ingredients.

CREAM OF CARROT SOUP

Recipe by Cherie.

Time: 35 minutes, plus 30 minutes to soak rice
Serves 4–6

Ingredients:

2 tablespoons extra-virgin olive oil
1 medium yellow onion, chopped
¾ teaspoon sea salt
2 pounds carrots, cut into one-inch pieces
5 cups vegetable stock
¼ cup cooked rice or raw cashews, soaked 30 minutes
2-inch piece of ginger, peeled and chopped
1 tablespoon lemon juice
Freshly ground black pepper, to taste

Instructions:

1. Heat a stock pot over medium heat, and add the olive oil. Add the onions and salt, sauteing for 5 minutes. Add the carrots and cover, cooking for another 5 minutes over medium heat.
2. Add the vegetable stock and the cooked rice or cashews to the pot and bring it to a boil. After the soup starts to boil, reduce the heat and simmer for 25 minutes.
3. Puree the soup in batches, being careful not to overfill the blender (a hot mess will happen!). Add the fresh chopped ginger into the soup as you puree. Stir in the lemon juice, and season with salt and pepper to taste.

Note: Add more stock at the end if you prefer your soup thinner.

GEORGE FOREMAN'S ROSEMARY-THYME MARINADE

This tangy marinade is great with fish or chicken. This is also Cherie's tribute to the late George Foreman, with whom she worked for thirteen years on QVC Grilling. George was committed to healthier eating and living, showing people healthy ways of making food.

Total time: 10 minutes
Makes about 1 cup marinade

Ingredients:

½ cup extra-virgin olive oil
¼ cup fresh lemon juice
2 garlic cloves, pressed
1 teaspoon dried thyme
1 teaspoon dried rosemary
½ teaspoon lemon zest

Instruction:

In a small bowl, combine all ingredients. Set aside until ready to use.

(From *Knock-Out-the-Fat Barbecue and Grilling Cookbook* by George Foreman and Cherie Calbom.)

CHERYL HINES'S WHITEFISH WITH LEMON CAPER SAUCE

(Cheryl Hines is an Award-Nominated actress and producer, and proud wife of the US Health and Human Services Secretary, Robert F. Kennedy Jr.)

Total time: 20 minutes
Serves 2

Ingredients:

2 (6-ounce) fillets firm wild-caught whitefish (branzino, snapper, sea bass, cod, mahimahi, sole, or flounder)

Sea salt, to taste
Freshly ground black pepper, to taste
2 tablespoons extra-virgin olive oil
1 medium shallot, minced, or 2 tablespoons minced onion
2 garlic cloves, minced
½ cup dry white wine or vegetable stock
Zest of 1 medium lemon
2 tablespoons lemon juice
2 tablespoons capers, rinsed
1 tablespoon minced parsley

Instructions:

1. Season the fish with salt and pepper on both sides.
2. Over medium heat, add olive oil and the fish to a frying pan. Cook on both sides until each side is browned. A light crust should form. Do not overcook the fish, and keep it moist. Carefully remove the fish from the pan and set aside.
3. In the same pan, add the shallot and garlic. Cook until tender and translucent.
4. Add the wine, lemon zest, and lemon juice.
5. Heat the sauce until it gently starts to bubble. Reduce heat.
6. Simmer the sauce for about 2 minutes or until it reduces a bit.
7. Add capers, parsley, salt, and pepper to taste.
8. Return the fish to the pan and cook for another 1 to 2 minutes or until the fish is warm. Serve warm, and spoon sauce over the fish before serving.

SOURDOUGH BREAD PIZZA WITH GRASS-FED BEEF AND BUFFALO MOZZARELLA

This recipe is by Dr. Josh Axe and Jordan Rubin from their book, *The Biblio Diet.*

Total time: 25 minutes
Serves 4

Ingredients:

2 tablespoons extra-virgin olive oil
1 pound grass-fed ground beef
I teaspoon sea salt
2 teaspoons Italian seasoning (oregano, basil, thyme)
8 slices bread (sourdough, einkorn, or sprouted is best)
1 cup tomato sauce (no added sugar)
8 slices raw buffalo mozzarella or provolone (8 ounces)

Instructions:

1. Preheat the oven to 375°F.
2. In a pan, heat the olive oil over medium heat. Add the ground beef, sea salt, and Italian seasoning, cooking until browned. Drain any excess fat.
3. Place the bread slices on a baking sheet. Spread tomato sauce evenly over each slice.
4. Top with the cooked beef and sliced cheese.
5. Bake for 10 minutes, or until the cheese is melted and bubbly.
6. Serve hot and enjoy! Makes plenty for leftovers.

REAL FOOD BAKED PASTA WITH TOMATO, HERBS, AND MOZZARELLA

by Kelly Ryerson, a.k.a. the Glyphosate Girl

Total time: 1 hour, 15 minutes
Serves 4

Ingredients:

- 2 tablespoons extra-virgin olive oil
- 1 garlic clove, minced
- 1 pinch red pepper flakes
- 1 pound lean ground beef or turkey
- 2 tablespoons tomato paste
- 1 (28-ounce) can of peeled Roma tomatoes, coarsely chopped
- 1 tablespoon dried oregano
- 1 teaspoon sea salt
- 1 teaspoon black pepper
- 12 ounces dry pasta (penne, fusilli, etc.—not long noodles)
- ¼ cup cream or half-and-half, optional
- 5 ounces fresh mozzarella
- ¼ cup fresh basil or parsley, chopped
- Grated Parmigiano Reggiano cheese

Instructions:

1. Preheat oven to 425°F.
2. Heat a pot of salted water and bring to a boil.
3. In a large frying pan, heat the oil until fragrant.
4. Add garlic and red pepper and sauté for 1 minute.
5. Add ground beef and cook until browned, using a fork or spoon to break up the meat as it cooks.
6. Once the meat is browned, add the tomato paste and cook for 2 minutes, until the tomato paste is incorporated into the meat. (If you are not using lean ground beef you may want to drain some of the rendered fat before adding the tomato paste.)

7. Add the chopped tomatoes, oregano, 1 teaspoon salt, and 1 teaspoon ground pepper.
8. Simmer, uncovered, as you prepare the pasta, at least 15 minutes.
9. Add dry pasta to the boiling water. Cook until slightly underdone (pasta will continue to cook in the oven).
10. When ready, drain the pasta and add to a large ceramic casserole dish.
11. Take the tomato sauce off the heat.
12. Add cream if using and the chopped parsley/basil. Stir to incorporate.
13. Add the sauce to the casserole dish with the pasta and stir to combine.
14. Taste the pasta and adjust salt and pepper as desired.
15. Thinly slice the mozzarella and layer on top.
16. Bake for 15 minutes—mozzarella should start to brown slightly.
17. Remove from the oven, allow to cool slightly, and serve with grated Parmigiano Reggiano cheese.

RECIPES WITH COCONUT OIL

Ways to Use Coconut Oil

Coconut oil can make a nice base for salad dressing when you melt it. Try a liquid coconut oil, like an MCT oil, that doesn't need to be melted. If you don't like the smell or taste of coconut oil, you can opt for a "refined" coconut oil, which means it's gone through an extra process to remove the smell and taste of coconut. It's still healthy. It is great for making cookies, cakes, cashew cheese, cashew ice cream, and cashew cheesecake. You can use butter-flavored coconut oil as a dairy butter substitute. It smells and tastes like butter, making it a great alternative. It is delicious on popcorn. You can also use coconut oil to scramble eggs and for sautéing.

WATERCRESS WEIGHT LOSS SOUP

Cherie's soup was very popular a few years ago, after it was featured as a cover story in *Women's World* magazine.

Total time: 20 minutes
Serves 4

Ingredients:

2 tablespoons coconut oil
2 cups sweet onion, diced
1 cup celery, diced
1 teaspoon sea salt, divided
4 medium zucchini, diced
4 cups vegetable broth
¼ cup unsweetened almond butter
2 cups watercress, chopped
2 teaspoons fresh lemon juice
Freshly ground pepper to taste

Instructions:

1. In a medium to large soup pot over medium heat, heat the oil and sauté the onion and celery with half of the salt for about 5 minutes, or until translucent. Add the zucchini and sauté for 3 minutes.
2. Add the vegetable broth and the other ½ teaspoon salt and pepper. Stir in the almond butter until well combined. Increase the heat to high, and bring to a boil. Reduce the heat to low, and simmer for about 5 minutes or until the zucchini is tender. Add the watercress and simmer for about 5 minutes. Turn off the heat, and let the soup cool slightly. Stir in the lemon juice.
3. If you want a creamy soup, pour it into a blender in batches and puree until smooth and creamy. Return the soup to the soup pot and warm over low heat.

SUPER-SPEEDY SUPPER

There are times when you need to prepare something healthy quickly. This recipe from Cherie is one of those dishes. There is nothing better than a juicy, crunchy salad to go with this supper, such as fresh tomatoes, cucumbers, radishes, green onions, and your favorite greens, dressed with lemon juice and a dash of olive oil or one of our vinaigrettes.

Total time: 20 minutes
Serves 4

Ingredients:

2 tablespoons virgin coconut oil
1 teaspoon cumin seeds
1 pound ground beef, buffalo, lamb, turkey, or chicken
½ medium cabbage, shredded
1 medium onion, chopped
1 teaspoon paprika

1 teaspoon nutmeg
1 tablespoon crushed garlic
2 tablespoons green olives, sliced
1 tablespoon finely chopped fresh parsley

Instructions:

1. Heat the oil in a pan and add the cumin seeds and ground meat. Stir for about 5 minutes.
2. Add the shredded cabbage, onion, paprika, nutmeg, crushed garlic, and olives. Mix well and stir-fry for another 5 minutes.
3. Garnish with parsley.

30-MINUTE CHICKEN NOODLE SOUP

Recipe by Liana.

Total time: 30 minutes
Serves 4

Ingredients:

1 tablespoon coconut oil
2 celery stalks, chopped
1 large carrot, chopped
1 brown onion, sliced
2 cloves garlic, minced
½ teaspoon dried basil
½ teaspoon dried oregano
½ teaspoon dried thyme
¼ teaspoon sea salt
¼ teaspoon pepper
56 ounces chicken broth
14 ounces vegetable broth
½ pound chicken strips

1 packet of your choice of noodles, either organic ramen or Explore Cuisine gluten-free rice or chickpea noodles.
Broccoli sprouts for serving

Instructions:

1. Place the oil, celery, carrot, onion, and garlic in a large pot and cook for 1 minute over medium-high heat. Pour in the rest of the ingredients, except for the noodles and broccoli sprouts.
2. Bring to a boil and allow to cook for 7 minutes.
3. Add the noodles and cook until they are done according to packet instructions.
4. When chicken and noodles are done, top with broccoli sprouts and serve.

Tip: You can make this plant-based for a veggie noodle soup if you like; just use vegetable broth and no chicken.

MINI CASHEW CHEESECAKES

This recipe contains healthy fats from the coconut oil. It's a "no guilt" treat! Regular cheesecakes are full of seed oils, refined sugars, and chemical ingredients. You can substitute almonds for cashews if you aren't into cashews; it just won't be as creamy. Recipe by Liana.

Total time: 10 minutes
Makes 20 mini cheesecakes

Ingredients:

3 cups cashew nuts
½ cup lemon juice
¾ cup maple syrup
¾ cup coconut oil
1 tablespoon pure vanilla extract
⅛ teaspoon sea salt

Instructions:

1. Soak cashews for at least 3 hours before. Put all the ingredients in a high-speed blender and whip until completely smooth.
2. Spoon 1 heaping tablespoon of the cheesecake mixture into each paper cupcake cup.
3. Set in the freezer for 6 minutes. Enjoy!

Tips:

- You'll need 20 small paper cupcake cups for this recipe. You can also make a regular-sized cheesecake.
- You will need a high-speed blender or food processor to make these creamy and without any chunks.
- Place a pecan, walnut, or macadamia nut on the top of each cupcake for decoration and texture.
- Keep these in the freezer or fridge until they set.

FEATHER-LIGHT COCONUT MACAROONS

Recipe by Cherie.

Total time: 40 minutes
Makes about 18 cookies

Ingredients:

1 tablespoon coconut oil
⅓ cup + 1 tablespoon whole wheat or gluten-free pastry flour, divided
3 egg whites
1 teaspoon pure vanilla extract
1 teaspoon stevia or monk fruit
½ cup dry unsweetened finely shredded coconut, divided
½ teaspoon baking soda
1 teaspoon lemon juice
2 tablespoons pure maple syrup

Instructions:

1. Preheat the oven to 300°F. Grease a cookie sheet with 1 tablespoon of coconut oil and sprinkle it with 1 tablespoon of flour.
2. Beat the egg whites until they are stiff enough to stand in peaks. Beat in the vanilla and the stevia.
3. In a separate bowl, combine ⅓ of the ½ cup shredded coconut, ⅓ cup flour, and baking soda. Mix well, and then add the lemon juice and the maple syrup. Mix again.
4. Carefully fold the egg whites into the coconut mixture, then drop by spoonful onto the prepared cookie sheet.
5. Bake at 300°F. Bake for 20 to 25 minutes, until golden. Then turn off the oven, remove the cookies from the cookie sheet, transfer them to a baker's rack, and let them set in the warm oven for another 20 minutes.
6. Sprinkle remaining coconut flakes on top of cookies.

PUMPKIN SPICE OATMEAL BALLS

Recipe by Cherie.

Total time: 15 minutes
Makes 24 balls

Ingredients:

1 (16-ounce) can unsweetened pumpkin puree
2 cups oats
1–2 cups chopped nuts such as pecans, almonds, or walnuts
½ cup coconut oil
½ cup pure maple syrup
2 tablespoons pumpkin pie spice
1 teaspoon pure vanilla extract
Pinch sea salt
½ cup unsweetened coconut flakes

Instructions:

1. In a medium bowl, mix pumpkin puree, oats, nuts, pumpkin pie spice, and salt, and mix well.
2. Combine coconut oil, vanilla, and maple syrup.
3. Pour the liquid mixture over the pumpkin, oats, and nuts mixture and combine well.
4. Scoop 1 to 2 tablespoons of the mixture, using your hands to roll into a ball.
5. Pour the coconut flakes onto a plate. Roll each ball in the coconut flakes.
6. Chill in the fridge for several hours or until ready to serve.

COCONUT LIME CUSTARD

Recipe by Cherie.

Time 20 minutes
Serves 4

Ingredients:

2 cups full-fat coconut milk
½ teaspoon sea salt
3 tablespoons grated lime zest
1 teaspoon pure vanilla extract
4 large pastured egg yolks
⅔ cup monk fruit or coconut sugar
¾ cup coconut oil

Instructions:

1. Combine the coconut milk, salt, lime zest, and vanilla in a saucepan. Heat on medium until barely boiling, about 5 minutes. Set aside to cool.
2. Beat the egg yolks and sweetener on medium-high speed for 3 to 5 minutes, or until thick. On low speed, slowly beat in the coconut oil until well blended, about 2 minutes.

3. Bring the coconut milk mixture back to a simmer over medium heat. Mix on medium speed, slowly adding the coconut milk; mix until well blended. Pour the custard back into the saucepan. Cook over medium heat, stirring constantly, until the custard coats the spatula, about 5 minutes.
4. Pour the custard into small bowls and set aside to completely cool.

FOOD BABE'S NO SUGAR GRANOLA BY VANI HARI

"I pretty much stopped buying granola from the store years ago. Most brands taste stale, processed, and overly sweet. After you make your own granola, it's really hard to go back to the packaged stuff! This granola is quick to make and contains no sugar or sweeteners at all. It has that delicious crunch along with naturally sweet coconut that makes it a savory and delicious topping for yogurt or as a snack by itself."

Total time: 20 minutes
Makes 4 to 6 servings

Ingredients:

- 2 cups unsweetened coconut flakes
- 1 cup mixed nuts of your choice, chopped (I like to use almonds, pecans, and walnuts)
- ½ cup pumpkin seeds (pepitas)
- ¼ cup sunflower seeds
- 2 tablespoons chia seeds
- 1 teaspoon ground cinnamon
- 1 teaspoon vanilla extract
- ¼ cup melted coconut oil

Instructions:

1. Heat the oven to 325° F.
2. Place all of the ingredients in a bowl and mix to combine.

3. Line a baking sheet with parchment paper. Spread the granola on a baking sheet and bake for 12 to 15 minutes. Let cool, then store in an airtight container for use during the week.

FIVE-SPICE SALMON

Bold, aromatic, and full of warmth, this five-spice salmon features a golden crust of turmeric, cumin, paprika, coriander, and a hint of cayenne. Pan-seared to perfection, it's crispy on the outside and tender, flaky on the inside. This is a simple yet show-stopping dish that brings exotic flavors to the weeknight table. Recipe by Maria Marlowe, The Acne Nutritionist.

Total time: 15 minutes
Serves 2

Ingredients:

2 (4- to 6-ounce) wild salmon fillets
Pinch of unrefined salt (Real Salt, pink salt, or Celtic salt)
Pinch of black pepper
¾ teaspoon turmeric
¾ teaspoon cumin powder
¾ teaspoon coriander powder
½ teaspoon paprika
¼ teaspoon cayenne powder
1 tablespoon unrefined coconut oil or unrefined avocado oil

Instructions:

1. Preheat the oven to 400°F. Also, on the stovetop, preheat a medium-sized skillet over medium heat for about 2 minutes.
2. Place the fish on a parchment-paper-lined baking sheet.
3. Sprinkle a pinch of salt and black pepper over the fish.
4. In a small bowl, combine the remaining spices and mix well. Spoon the spices over the fish and use the back of the spoon to press it in, until the pink flesh is entirely coated with the spices, and you can't see any pink.

5. Once your pan is hot enough, add the oil, and then place the fillets coated-side down in the pan.
6. Cook for about 2½ minutes, until the spice mixture forms a nicely browned crust. Flip the fillets (they should release easily) and cook for another 2 minutes. Then, transfer to the baking sheet and put in the oven to finish cooking, 4 to 8 minutes depending on thickness and how well done you'd like it. Less for a thinner cut, more for a thicker cut. It should reach an internal temperature of 145°F.

RECIPES WITH MCT OIL

Ways to Use MCT Oil

MCT oil delivers primarily caprylic (C8) and capric (C10) acids. It is considered flavorless and odorless, making it easy to mix into various foods and beverages without altering their taste. It is a neutral oil that can be added to coffee, smoothies, salad dressings, and sauces, and used for mid-temperature cooking.

LIANA'S OG 3-HOUR CHICKEN BONE BROTH NOODLE SOUP

This recipe is great for freezing and meal prepping. I (Liana) usually cook a batch and eat it once daily for three days, and then freeze the other four servings in Tupperware. Reheat in a covered pot on the stove to retain moisture. Do not use a microwave, as you will kill all the nutrients.

Total time: 3 hours
Makes 7–9 bowls

Ingredients:

For the Broth:

1 whole organic pasture-raised chicken (take out the giblets from inside the chicken)
1½ gallons filtered water
7 garlic cloves
3 thumb-size pieces of ginger, diced
1 thumb-size piece of turmeric, diced, or 1 teaspoon ground turmeric
1 whole onion, sliced
3 celery stalks, chopped
1 tablespoon Redmond Real Salt Organic Seasoning
1 teaspoon black pepper
1 tablespoon thyme
1 tablespoon oregano

1 lemon, peeled and seeded (make sure the seeds are out or your soup will be bitter!)
2 tablespoons olive oil
2 tablespoons MCT oil

For the Soup:

Chicken meat (from the boiled chicken)
4 carrots, sliced
1 cup green beans, trimmed
1 head broccoli, chopped into bite-size pieces
3 celery stalks, chopped
Noodles of your choice (rice, chickpea, or red lentil), optional

Instructions:

1. In a large pot add the chicken and water.
2. Add garlic, ginger, turmeric, onion, celery, salt, pepper, thyme, oregano, peeled lemon, olive oil, and MCT oil.
3. Bring to a boil, then reduce to a high simmer, place a lid on top, and cook for 2 hours. Check occasionally and add more water as needed.
4. After 2 hours, turn off the heat and allow soup to cool with lid on, about 30 minutes. Remove the chicken from the pot. Carefully separate the meat from the bones.
5. Return the chicken meat to the pot and discard the bones (or save for other uses).
6. Add sliced carrots, green beans, broccoli, and celery to the pot. You can either simmer for 10 to 15 minutes until the vegetables are tender, or just keep the vegetables raw and start putting them in Tupperware, and when you reheat them the vegetables will cook then.
7. Stir in cooked noodles, if using, just before serving to heat through.
8. Ladle into bowls and enjoy the comforting warmth of this nutrient-packed chicken noodle soup.

Tip: For added flavor, sprinkle with fresh parsley or a squeeze of lemon juice before serving.

COMFORTING CREAMY TOMATO SOUP

(Recipe by Liana.)

Total time: 30 minutes
Serves 3

Ingredients:

28-ounce can whole tomatoes, in juice
5 large tomatoes
15 cherry tomatoes
8 cups water
1 celery stalk, coarsely chopped
¼ small onion, coarsely chopped
1 garlic clove
1 teaspoon dried parsley
1 teaspoon dried thyme
1 bay leaf
1 tablespoon honey
1 fresh lemon juice
¼ teaspoon salt
¼ teaspoon black pepper
2 tablespoons MCT oil
2 tablespoons olive oil
¼ cup organic cream or coconut cream, optional
¼ cup organic cheese shreds or vegan shreds, optional

Instructions:

1. Puree all ingredients in a blender until smooth. Taste. Season with more salt and pepper, if desired.
2. Add the raw smooth soup blend to a pot and bring to a boil. Boil for 10 minutes and then reduce heat and simmer for another 10 minutes. Serve with fresh herbs and avocado slices.

Tips: You can enjoy this soup raw if you like, or cook it! That's the beauty of this soup. This also can be used as a sauce when cooking ground beef, spaghetti, lasagna, or any other recipe that calls for "pasta sauce."

CHOCOLATE SUPERFOOD BALLS

These chocolate balls aren't just a recipe—they're a turning point. They were the very first recipe Liana ever made when she chose to break her addiction to refined sugar when she started The Earth Diet in 2009. Made with raw cacao, a true superfood known for its antioxidant content and natural energy boost, these chocolate balls satisfy cravings while nourishing the body. Hemp seeds provide easily assimilated plant-based protein, MCT oil offers clean fuel for the brain, and a touch of almond oil brings warmth and depth of flavor. A key ingredient is apricot seed meal, which naturally contains B17 (amygdalin). Liana learned about apricot seeds through John Richardson, who carries on the legacy of his father, a medical doctor who treated and educated others on their traditional use. Liana recommends 5–10 apricot seeds per day as part of a mindful lifestyle, and because the seeds are quite bitter, these chocolate balls offer a fun, sweet way to enjoy them.

Total time: 10 minutes
Makes 12 balls

Ingredients:

1 cup almond flour
¼ cup raw cacao powder
3 tablespoons honey or maple syrup
2 tablespoons RNC apricot seed meal
1 tablespoon MCT oil
3 tablespoons hemp seeds
⅛ teaspoon almond oil
Pinch of Real Salt

Instructions:

Mix all ingredients into a bowl until well combined. Add a dash of water to the mixture if dry. It should be moist enough to roll into balls and hold well.

Pro tips:

- Roll in shredded coconut.
- Add in some food-grade essential oils like cinnamon, orange, or peppermint for refreshing flavors.

RECIPES WITH AVOCADO OIL

Ways to Use Avocado Oil

Avocado oil is very versatile for cooking due to its mild buttery flavor with grassy undertones and high smoke point. It enhances dishes rather than overwhelming them. Avocado oil is ideal for searing, frying, grilling, and baking, as well as for marinades, salad dressings, and as a butter substitute in baked goods.

WALNUT-CRUSTED CHICKEN TENDERS

This was one of the very first recipes I ever created to replace every time I had a craving for KFC fried chicken. The crust is golden, crunchy, and so delicious with the tender chicken inside. You can bake, fry, or air-fry these. Recipe by Liana.

Total time: 20–30 minutes, depending on your cooking method
Serves 4

Ingredients:

- ⅓ cup walnut meal
- ½ cup almond flour
- 1½ tablespoons turmeric powder
- ¼ teaspoon sea salt
- ¼ teaspoon black pepper
- 2 eggs
- 1 pound boneless, skinless chicken breasts
- ¾ cup + 1 tablespoon extra-virgin coconut oil, divided
- 1 handful of broccoli sprouts, for garnish

Instructions:

1. Preheat the oven to 450°F if you are using the baking method.
2. Add the walnut meal, almond flour, turmeric, salt, and pepper to a bowl and mix until well combined.

3. Beat the eggs in a separate bowl.
4. Cut the chicken into tenders.
5. Dip the tenders into the egg and then into the breading, turning until they're coated well on all sides.
6. Cook according to your preferred method, below.
7. Serve garnished with a sprinkle of broccoli sprouts and a side salad.

Cooking methods

Bake (with avocado oil)

1. Preheat oven to 450°F. Brush or spray baking sheet with avocado oil.
2. Place chicken on sheet; lightly oil the top. Bake for 15 to 20 minutes.

Panfry (with coconut oil)

1. In skillet, heat coconut oil.
2. Add chicken and cook 5 to 6 minutes per side.

Air Fry (with avocado oil spray)

1. Preheat air fryer to 375°F. Spray the basket with avocado oil.
2. Air fry 10 minutes; flip; cook 6 to 8 minutes more.

To Serve

Plate chicken and garnish with chopped fresh parsley and sauce.

BLACK BEAN, CORN, AND QUINOA SALAD

Recipe by Cherie.

Total time: 35 minutes
Serves 6

Ingredients:

2 cups organic free-range chicken or vegetable broth
1 cup uncooked quinoa
1 cup organic corn, fresh or frozen
1 tablespoon lime juice

Zest of 1 lime
1 teaspoon red wine vinegar
½ teaspoon ground cumin
2 tablespoons avocado oil
1 (15-ounce) can black beans, drained
1 small red bell pepper, seeded and chopped
1 small red onion, finely chopped
½ cup chopped fresh cilantro
Sea salt and ground black pepper to taste

Instructions:

1. Bring broth to a boil in a saucepan. Stir in quinoa. Reduce heat to low; simmer, covered, until liquid is absorbed, 15 to 20 minutes. Remove the quinoa from the heat and stir in the corn. Let stand, covered, until corn is warmed, about 5 minutes.
2. Combine lime juice in a large bowl with red wine vinegar, lime zest, and cumin. Whisk in avocado oil. Add black beans, red bell pepper, onion, and cilantro. Season with salt and pepper. Stir in quinoa and corn.
3. Chill until ready to serve.

BEET BROWNIES

Recipe by Cherie.

Total time: 35 minutes
Serves 8

Ingredients:

½ cup mashed organic (non-GMO) silken tofu (medium firmness)
½ cup beet juice, plant milk, or water
½ cup pure maple syrup or coconut syrup
½ cup almond oil
1 teaspoon pure vanilla extract

½ cup garbanzo flour
½ cup cocoa powder
1½ teaspoons baking powder
½ cup grated beets or beet pulp (leftover from juicing)
½ cup sugar-free or stevia-sweetened chocolate chips
½ cup chopped nuts

Instructions:

1. Combine tofu, beet juice, maple syrup, almond oil, and vanilla in a blender or with a mixer and blend until smooth and creamy. In a mixing bowl, sift together flour, cocoa, and baking powder. Mix well. Add grated beets or beet puree, and mix to distribute evenly throughout the flour. Then stir in chocolate chips and nuts. Add the blended mixture to the flour mixture.
2. Mix well to combine ingredients and form a batter. Transfer the batter into an 8 × 8-inch baking pan that has been generously oiled and floured. Bake at 350°F for about 25 minutes or until firm to the touch. Let it cool in the pan before slicing and removing.

AVOCADO CHOCOLATE CHIP COOKIES

Recipe by Cherie.

Total time: 35 minutes
Makes 14 cookies

Ingredients:

⅓ cup avocado oil
½ cup monk fruit or coconut sugar
⅔ cup mashed avocado
2 large free-range eggs
½ teaspoon sea salt
1 teaspoon lemon juice
2 cups almond flour

⅓ cup coconut flour; add more if needed

⅔ cup unsweetened or stevia-sweetened chocolate chips

Instructions:

1. Preheat oven to 350°F.
2. Mix oil, monk fruit, salt, and mashed avocado. Beat for 1 to 2 minutes.
3. Add eggs and continue mixing.
4. Add lemon juice.
5. Stir in flour until well combined and smooth but not sticky. Last, stir in chocolate chips. You should be able to shape the batter in your hands; if it's sticky, add more coconut flour (about 2 tablespoons).
6. Let the cookie dough chill in the fridge for 5 to 10 minutes, or until cool.
7. Remove the cookie dough from the fridge and, using a cookie scoop or about 2 tablespoons of dough, drop batter onto a greased cookie sheet so that the cookies are at least 1 inch apart.
8. Bake the cookies at 350°F for about 15 minutes or until slightly golden on the top.
9. Let cool completely before serving.

HEALING STRONG'S MOCK TUNA SALAD

Recipe from Healing Strong, a nonprofit organization that walks alongside those facing cancer and other chronic illnesses, offering hope, encouragement, and community, while teaching strategies that help empower each person to journey toward healing with courage, support, and purpose. Visit Healing Strong at https://healingstrong.org/.

Total time: 20 minutes
Serves 4

Ingredients:

1 can organic chickpeas, drained

1 tablespoon avocado oil

½ avocado, mashed
½ cup diced celery
¼ cup diced onion
1 tablespoon dill pickle relish (use Bubbies fermented pickles for added probiotic benefits)
1 tablespoon lemon juice
1 teaspoon sea salt
½ teaspoon dulse or other seaweed sprinkle

Instructions:

1. Place all ingredients in the bowl of a food processor and pulse until it reaches the consistency of tuna salad. Do not over-blend.
2. If the mixture seems too dry, you can add more liquid (pickle juice, lemon juice, or avocado oil), or a mixture of any or all.

Tips: You can serve this on sliced tomatoes, on top of a salad, or in a lettuce leaf like a wrap.

If you want a vegan tuna melt using a healthy bread like Ezekiel, note that vegan dairy substitutes often use soy; we recommend finding brands that use nuts such as cashews instead of soy.

RECIPES WITH MACADAMIA NUT OIL

Ways to Use Macadamia Nut Oil

Because macadamia nut oil has a mild, buttery flavor, it is great for baked goods and salad dressings. It is good for frying, baking, roasting, and making salad dressings and marinades. Due to its high smoke point, it is suitable for high-heat cooking methods such as frying and grilling.

MACADAMIA NUT SALAD

Recipe by Cherie.

Total time: 35 minutes
Serves 4–6

Ingredients:

Salad

- ¾ cup macadamia nuts
- 1 tablespoon coconut aminos
- 2–3 teaspoons ginger, finely grated
- 1 cup brown rice
- 1 cup quinoa
- 1½ cups cold water
- 1 bunch of asparagus
- 2 beets
- 1 medium carrot
- 1 teaspoon coriander
- ½ cup micro sprouts

Dressing

- 1 tablespoon ginger, finely grated
- 1 tablespoon coconut aminos
- 1 tablespoon apple cider vinegar
- 1 tablespoon monk fruit
- ¼ cup macadamia nut oil

Instructions:

1. Preheat oven to 350°F. Place the macadamia nuts in a bowl and stir in the coconut aminos and ginger until completely coated. Scatter over a baking sheet and bake for 10 minutes. Allow nuts to cool before coarsely chopping. Set aside.
2. In salted boiling water, cook the rice until tender. Drain and set aside. Rinse the quinoa in cold water; drain. Add 1½ cups of cold water to a saucepan and bring to a boil. Reduce the heat to low, cover, and cook 15 minutes. Next, let it stand for 12 minutes. Remove the lid and fluff the grains with a fork to separate. Set aside.
3. Cut the bottom quarter off the asparagus. (You can save the stems for juicing.) Lightly steam for 5 minutes.
4. Using tongs, remove the spears; rinse under cold water. Cut spears into thirds and set aside. Grate the beets and carrot. Combine the asparagus with the other vegetables and coriander and set aside.
5. Make the dressing by shaking vigorously in a jar. Divide the dressing into thirds, then evenly distribute it over the brown rice, quinoa, and vegetables. Stir to combine. Layer it on a platter, and sprinkle with ginger and coconut aminos, macadamia nuts, and micro sprouts. Serve immediately.

KETO-FRIENDLY, IMMUNITY-BOOSTING FAT FLUSH SOUP

This is a brand-new version of Ann Louise Gittleman's famous Fat Flush Soup, which balances immune support with keto-friendly ingredients! Recipe by Anne Louise Gittleman, PhD in holistic nutrition and national best-selling author of *Radical Metabolism* and *Radical Longevity,* along with the *New York Times* bestseller *Fat Flush.*

Total time: 25 minutes
Makes 12–14 cups

Ingredients:

2 tablespoons macadamia nut oil
1 pound chopped chicken breast, lean ground turkey or grass-fed ground beef
1 large onion, diced
3 garlic cloves, minced
3 cups sliced fresh or frozen mixed mushrooms (containing shiitake)
2 teaspoons fresh thyme (or 1 teaspoon dried thyme)
2 tablespoons curry powder
4 cups chicken, turkey or beef bone broth (preferably homemade for added nutrients)
1 medium zucchini, cut to your preference
1 medium yellow squash, cut to your preference
1 can (14 ounces) full-fat coconut cream
⅓ cup parsley, chopped (save a few pinches for garnish)
1 teaspoon sea salt

Instructions:

1. Heat oil in a large pot over medium heat.
2. Add your preferred protein and cook until browned and fully cooked through (5 to 7 minutes). If you chose ground beef as your protein, drain off all drippings, and return to pot. If you find there is not enough oil left in pot after draining off drippings, add 1 tablespoon macadamia nut oil and continue with instructions.
3. Add to pot diced onion and minced garlic, and sauté for 2 to 3 minutes until softened, transparent, and fragrant.
4. Stir in sliced mushrooms, thyme, and curry, and cook for an additional 2 to 3 minutes. Pour in bone broth and bring the soup to a boil.
5. Add zucchini, yellow squash, and coconut cream.
6. Lower the heat and let the soup simmer for 15 to 20 minutes, or until vegetables are tender.

7. Add chopped parsley to soup in the last 5 minutes; save some to garnish with as well.
8. Season with salt, to taste. Adjust seasonings as preferred.
9. Serve warm and enjoy the immune-boosting, Fat Flush benefits!

RECIPE WITH SESAME SEED OIL

Ways to Use Sesame Seed Oil

Sesame seed oil gives a rich, nutty flavor to a variety of recipes, making it a versatile ingredient in cooking. It is commonly used in stir-fries, dressings, marinades, soups, broths, and savory dishes.

THAI CHICKEN SUPER SALAD

Recipe by Dr. Cate Shanahan. "I love the bright, bold, blend of savory, fruity, and nutty flavors. It doesn't require mayo, so it's lighter and less filling than the typical mayo-based chicken salad. As with all my super salads, I usually make this my main dinner dish, and make a big pile of it."

Total time: 10–15 minutes
Serves 1

Ingredients:

Salad

5–6 ounces chopped leftover chicken breast (or turkey)
1 medium carrot, chopped fine
1 large celery stalk or several very small pieces of celery heart, and the leaves chopped fine, totaling about ½ cup
¾ scallion, chopped fine, about 1 tablespoon

Dressing

2 tablespoons sesame seed oil
1–1½ tablespoons lime/lemon juice
1½ teaspoons prepared brown mustard
½ teaspoon fish sauce
1 teaspoon toasted sesame seeds

Combine chicken, carrot, celery, and scallion in salad bowl. Mix all dressing ingredients and drizzle over the top of the salad. Stir together and serve.

RECIPES WITH GRASS-FED BUTTER

Ways to Use Butter

Butter brings rich creaminess to a wide range of dishes and is one of the most versatile ingredients in the kitchen. It enhances both flavor and texture, making it ideal for pansearing and basting meats, enriching rice and pasta, or melting over freshly cooked vegetables. It's also coveted in pie crusts and pastries, where it creates the tender, flaky layers we love. And of course, it's perfect simply spread on warm toast or muffins. Because butter begins to burn at around 302 °F, it's best suited for low to moderate temperature cooking.

BULLETPROOF COFFEE

Recipe by Cherie.

Total time: 5 minutes
Serves 1–2

Ingredients:

1 tablespoon unsalted grass-fed butter
1 teaspoon coconut oil
16 ounces fresh-brewed coffee
Dash of sea salt
Dash of cinnamon
Dash of nutmeg

Instructions:

1. Mix the butter and coconut oil into the coffee. Sprinkle the salt, cinnamon, and nutmeg on top and stir.

BUTTERY POPCORN

Recipe by Cherie.

Total time: 10 minutes
Serves: 2

Enjoy your own healthy popcorn while watching movies and avoid the stuff with seed oils, dyes, and chemicals.

Ingredients:

½ cup popcorn kernels
3 tablespoons grass-fed butter
3 tablespoons coconut oil
Sea salt to taste

Instructions:

1. Pop the corn in an air popper or kettle.
2. Melt the butter and coconut oil. Mix well.
3. Pour over the popcorn, and sprinkle with sea salt.
4. Add more salt as desired.

CHERIE'S LEMON CHICKEN STIR-FRY WITH ASPARAGUS AND CHERRY TOMATOES

This dish can be served alone or accompanied by whole-grain brown, black, or jade pearl rice.

Total time: 25 minutes
Serves 2

Ingredients:

2 chicken breasts cut into bite-size pieces
1 cup cherry tomatoes
1 cup chopped asparagus
2–3 tablespoons butter

Lemon Garlic Marinade

Juice and zest of 1 lemon
3 garlic cloves, minced
½ cup coconut oil or olive oil
1 tablespoon dried oregano
½ teaspoon sea salt
½ teaspoon ground pepper
1 cup of cooked whole-grain rice

Instructions:

1. Mix all marinade ingredients in a small bowl with a whisk until well combined. Place the chicken pieces into a medium bowl and pour the marinade over them.
2. Marinate for 1 hour.
3. In a medium saucepan, cook the rest of the ingredients until chicken is done, about 15 minutes.
4. Serve over whole-grain rice as desired.

COUNTRY-STYLE BUTTER PIECRUST

Grass-fed butter gives a piecrust a rich flavor and a tender, flaky texture. Recipe by Cherie.

Total time: 1 hour
Makes 1 piecrust

Ingredients:

1¼ cups organic unbleached all-purpose flour
1 teaspoon sea salt
½ cup butter, chilled and cut into small pieces
¼ cup purified ice water, as needed

Instructions:

1. Combine flour and salt in a large bowl.

2. Add chilled butter to the flour mixture, and use a pastry blender or your fingers to mix it in until it resembles coarse crumbs.
3. Slowly add the ice water, 1 tablespoon at a time, and mix until the dough comes together. Be careful not to overwork the dough.
4. Shape the dough into a disk. Wrap in plastic and refrigerate for 30 minutes.
5. Roll the dough on a floured surface to fit your pie dish. Add your desired filling, then bake according to the directions.

GLUTEN-FREE SHORTBREAD COOKIES

Recipe by Cherie.

Total time: 1 hour, 25 minutes
Makes 24 cookies

Ingredients:

2½ cups blanched almond flour
¼ teaspoon sea salt
¼ teaspoon baking soda
1 cup toasted pecans, chopped
5 tablespoons coconut nectar
½ cup salted grass-fed butter
1 tablespoon pure vanilla extract

Instructions:

1. Preheat oven to 350°F.
2. Combine flour, salt, baking soda, and pecans in a large bowl.
3. Mix coconut nectar, butter, and vanilla in a small bowl.
4. Combine wet ingredients with dry.
5. Place the dough on a cutting board that is covered with parchment paper and form into a log about 2½ inches in diameter. Wrap log with the parchment paper.
6. Place in the freezer for 1 hour, or until firm, and then unwrap.

7. Cut into ¼-inch slices.
8. Place slices on a parchment-paper-lined baking sheet. Bake 7 to 10 minutes, or until golden brown.
9. Cool and enjoy!

CHERIE'S BEST-EVER GARLIC BUTTER MASHED POTATOES

Total time: 15–20 minutes
Serves 6

Ingredients:

20–30 unpeeled garlic cloves
8 tablespoons grass-fed butter, divided
2 tablespoons organic all-purpose flour or gluten-free flour such as garbanzo bean flour
1 cup grass-fed whole milk or unsweetened plant milk
2½ pounds russet potatoes, peeled and cut into 1-inch pieces
¼ cup grass-fed heavy cream (optional)
Sea salt and ground white pepper, to taste
¼ cup finely chopped parsley leaves

Instructions:

1. In a small pot, bring water to a boil. Then add the garlic cloves and boil for 2 minutes; drain and peel.
2. Return the garlic cloves to the pan, add 4 tablespoons of butter, and cook on low until the garlic is soft, 15 to 20 minutes.
3. Stir in the flour and add the milk. Stir well and cook until bubbling, 3 to 4 minutes.
4. Use an immersion blender or a regular blender and puree. Set aside.
5. Place potatoes in a pot and bring to a boil. Reduce the heat to a simmer until soft, about 15 minutes.

6. Drain the potatoes, then rice them or mash them with a potato masher until fine.
7. Turn the heat to medium-low and stir in the remaining butter, garlic-butter sauce, cream (if using), salt, and pepper. With a hand mixer, combine all ingredients until well blended. Heat for 2 minutes. Sprinkle with parsley and serve.

MOMMA MANDY'S WHITE BEAN CHICKEN CHILI

Contributed by Leah Wilson, cofounder of Stand for Health Freedom and author of two foundational resources *The Vaccine Decision and Reclaim Vitality: A Guide to Exit Conventional Medicine and Live Naturally.* "This recipe is a staple in our house. It is a cozy, gently herby white chili that's nourishing, simple, and crowd-pleasing—perfect for a family dinner or easy hosting night."

Total time: 1½ hours plus 15 minutes of prep time
Serves; 6

Ingredients:

¼ cup organic (preferably raw) butter
1 cup chopped organic yellow onion
3 cloves organic garlic, minced
4 cups shredded cooked chicken breast
32 ounces organic great northern beans, drained and rinsed
1 small jar diced organic green chilies
½ cup salsa verde
1 tablespoon organic basil
3–6 cups organic chicken bone broth (adjust for desired thickness)
1 teaspoon sea salt (adjust to taste)

Optional Toppings:

Fresh organic cilantro, chopped
Shredded raw cheddar cheese

Diced avocado
Sour cream
Diced red onion
Crunchy tortilla chips made with no seed oils

Instructions:

1. In a large pot, melt the butter over medium heat.
2. Add the chopped onion and garlic. Sauté until soft and golden, 5 to 7 minutes.
3. Stir in the shredded chicken, beans, green chilies, salsa verde, basil, and 3 cups of bone broth.
4. Bring to a gentle simmer, then reduce heat to medium-low.
5. Cook uncovered for 30 to 40 minutes, stirring occasionally. Add additional bone broth as needed until thick—but not too thick.
6. Taste and add salt if desired.
7. Serve in individual bowls and top with your favorite toppings.

Serving Tip: This chili thickens even more as it sits, making leftovers especially delicious the next day. Add a splash of bone broth when reheating to loosen it up. Warm, comforting, and full of simple goodness

MARLA MAPLES'S GLUTEN-FREE COCONUT SUGAR PECAN PIE

"A true southern Thanksgiving tradition that I made healthier along the way as I learned!"

Total time: 45 minutes
Serves 4–8

Ingredients:

1 cup organic coconut sugar
3 tablespoons melted room-temperature grass-fed butter
3 room-temperature eggs

¾ cup organic maple syrup
¼–½ teaspoon sea salt
1 teaspoon vanilla extract
2 cups halved pecans, divided
1 gluten-free piecrust, unbaked

Instructions:

1. Mix the organic coconut sugar, butter, eggs, maple syrup, salt, and vanilla well with a whisk.
2. Stir in 1 cup of halved pecans.
3. Lay the remaining 1 cup of pecans on the bottom of the unbaked piecrust, then pour in the batter.
4. Bake at 400°F for 20 minutes, then lower the temperature to 350°F and bake for another 30 minutes.
5. Let cool before serving and enjoy with family and friends!

PALEO HUMMINGBIRD MUFFINS (MADE WITH REAL-FOOD FATS)

These muffins taste like a tropical banana-pineapple cake, but they're made with simple, nourishing ingredients and real fats your body knows what to do with.

Instead of industrial seed oils, I chose butter (or coconut oil/avocado oil) as an easy swap because these fats are naturally occurring, minimally processed, and stable when heated. They help keep you satisfied and support hormones, brain function, and energy—without relying on ultra-processed oils. Recipe by Lexi Noel, Health Coach and one of the founders of MAHA Girls.

Total time: 45 minutes
Makes 12 muffins

Ingredients:

1½ cups mashed very ripe bananas (about 4)

1 (8-ounce) can crushed pineapple, well-drained and squeezed (about ⅓ cup after draining)
¾ cup coconut sugar (or unrefined sugar of choice)
½ cup unsalted butter, melted (or coconut oil for dairy-free)
¼ cup whole milk (or coconut/almond milk if desired)
1 large egg
1½ cups organic all-purpose flour
1 teaspoon cinnamon
¼ teaspoon nutmeg
1½ teaspoons baking soda
1 teaspoon sea salt
½ cup pecans, chopped and toasted

Instructions:

1. Preheat oven to 350°F. Line a 12-cup muffin pan or grease lightly.
2. In a bowl, stir together bananas, pineapple, coconut sugar, melted butter, milk, and egg.
3. In another bowl, whisk flour, cinnamon, nutmeg, baking soda, and salt.
4. Make a well in the center and pour in the wet mixture. Stir gently until just combined.
5. Fold in pecans.
6. Fill muffin cups about ¾ full.
7. Bake for 20 to 25 minutes, until a toothpick comes out clean.
8. Cool for 15 minutes, then remove to a rack to finish cooling.
9. Store wrapped at room temperature for 2 days, or freeze for up to 2 months.

RECIPES WITH GHEE

Ways to Use Ghee

Rich, nutty, and caramel-like are the descriptors for ghee. You can swap it for butter or oil in many recipes. Scramble eggs or cook pancakes in ghee. Spread it on sourdough bread or a bagel. Use it to sauté vegetables and seafood, or to deep-fry fritters. Stir it into hot cereal or brush it over grilled chicken. Ghee is also great for baking, such as shortbread or cake.

ANTI-INFLAMMATORY GOLDEN MILK

Recipe by Cherie.

Total time: 5 minutes
Serves 1

Ingredients:

1 cup plant milk, or grass-fed dairy
1 tablespoon grated ginger
1 teaspoon monk fruit or a few drops of liquid stevia
1 teaspoon ghee
½ teaspoon ground turmeric
½ teaspoon ground cinnamon
⅛ teaspoon ground black pepper

Instructions:

1. Combine all the ingredients in a small saucepan and whisk until well combined.
2. Stir occasionally over medium heat for 5 to 10 minutes.
3. Strain out the ginger and serve.

DR. LAKE'S PUMPKIN PANCAKES

Total time: 25 minutes
Makes 8–10 pancakes

Ingredients:

2 cups einkorn flour
2 teaspoons baking powder
1 teaspoon baking soda
1 teaspoon cinnamon
½ teaspoon nutmeg
½ teaspoon sea salt
1½ cups raw milk (or full-fat coconut milk)
1 cup organic pumpkin puree
1 large egg, pastured
2 tablespoons melted grass-fed butter or ghee
¼ cup pure maple syrup

Instructions:

1. In a large bowl, whisk together the flour, baking powder, baking soda, cinnamon, nutmeg, and salt. In a separate bowl, combine the milk, pumpkin puree, egg, butter, and maple syrup. Pour the wet mixture into the dry ingredients and whisk until smooth. If the batter is very thick, add 1 to 2 tablespoons of milk to reach a pourable consistency.
2. Heat a skillet over medium heat and lightly grease with butter or tallow. Pour ¼ to ½ cup of batter per pancake onto the skillet. Cook until small bubbles form and pop on the surface, then flip and cook until golden brown on the second side.
3. Serve warm with butter and pure maple syrup.

DR. WILL COLE'S SKILLET EGGS WITH SPINACH

This nourishing egg recipe is an excellent way to break your fast with 17 g of protein, 300 calories, 24 g of fat including 11.6 g of saturated fat, and just 4 g of net carbs per serving. From *Intuitive Fasting* by Dr. Will Cole, leading functional medicine expert and *New York Times* bestselling author.

Total time: 7 minutes
Serves 2

Ingredients:

2 tablespoons ghee
2 teaspoons fresh lemon juice
1 teaspoon chili powder
9 ounces (about 5½ cups) fresh spinach
¼ teaspoon sea salt
4 large eggs
½ cup chopped tomatoes
Black pepper to taste

Instructions:

1. In a large skillet, heat the ghee over medium-high heat. When ghee has melted, remove 1 tablespoon and place in a small bowl with the lemon juice and chili powder. Set aside.
2. To the remaining ghee in the skillet, add the spinach and ¼ teaspoon salt; cook 1 minute until just beginning to wilt, using two utensils to toss as you would a stir-fry.
3. Make four wells in the spinach. Carefully break 1 egg into each well. Cook for 3 to 4 minutes or until the egg whites are set.
4. Remove from heat. Drizzle with the reserved ghee mixture, sprinkle with tomatoes, and season lightly with salt and pepper to taste.

DR. JESS'S GOLDEN ANTI-INFLAMMATORY RICE BOWLS WITH HERBY LEMON CHICKEN

This is one of those meals that looks indulgent but quietly supports your liver, mitochondria, hormones, and nervous system. This recipe combines mineral-rich spices, clean fats, quality protein, and gentle acids that aid digestion rather than stress it.

Turmeric + fat + pepper = enhanced anti-inflammatory signaling. Basmati is gentler on insulin than most rices, and bone broth supports gut lining and mineral status.

Oregano and garlic are antimicrobial (hello gut health), lemon and apple cider vinegar support bile flow, and yogurt tenderizes the protein without wrecking digestion.

(By Dr. Jess Peatross, functional medicine doctor and supplement formulator, drjessmd.com.)

Total time: 30–40 minutes
Serves 4–6

Ingredients:

For the Lemon-Herb Chicken (Protein and Liver Support)

4 organic garlic cloves, crushed
2 tablespoons fresh lemon juice
1 tablespoon raw apple cider vinegar (instead of white wine vinegar)
1 tablespoon extra-virgin olive oil
2 tablespoons organic dried oregano
2 tablespoons full-fat A2 Greek yogurt (or coconut yogurt if dairy-free)
1 teaspoon sea salt
1 teaspoon organic smoked paprika
1 teaspoon ground cumin
1 pound pasture-raised, boneless, skinless chicken thighs, diced

Golden Rice (Inflammation-Calming Base)

2 tablespoons grass-fed butter or ghee
1 teaspoon organic ground turmeric
1 teaspoon organic ground cumin
1½ cups organic basmati rice (lower arsenic, easier on blood sugar)
2½ cups homemade bone broth or clean organic chicken stock
½ teaspoon unrefined sea salt
Freshly cracked black pepper (activates curcumin absorption)

For the Fresh Toppings (Detox and Mineral Boost)

Ingredients:

1 organic cucumber, diced
7 ounces organic cherry tomatoes, quartered
2 teaspoons sumac (antioxidant and digestion support)
½ teaspoon sea salt
Black pepper
½ cup clean tzatziki (preferably homemade with A2 yogurt or coconut yogurt)
A handful of fresh flat-leaf parsley (natural detoxifier)
Sourdough or grain-free flatbreads (optional)

Instructions:

Marinate the Chicken

1. Preheat oven to 480°F.
2. In a bowl or lidded container, combine garlic, lemon juice, apple cider vinegar, olive oil, oregano, yogurt, salt, smoked paprika, and cumin. Mix well, then toss in the chicken until fully coated.

Tip: Marinate for up to 24 hours—this improves digestibility and reduces inflammatory by-products during cooking.

Make the Golden Rice

1. Heat a large pot over medium heat. Melt butter, then add turmeric and cumin. Cook until fragrant (about 1 minute).
2. Add rice and stir to coat in the spices and fat. Toast gently for 2 to 3 minutes.
3. Pour in bone broth. Add salt and a generous grind of black pepper.

Simmer the Rice

1. Bring to a boil, then reduce heat to low, cover, and cook 15 minutes undisturbed.
2. Remove from heat and let steam (lid on) for 10 more minutes. This keeps the rice fluffy and blood sugar–friendly.

Roast the Chicken

1. Line a baking tray with unbleached parchment paper. Spread chicken in a single layer.
2. Roast for 20 minutes, until golden and lightly charred at the edges (that flavor comes without frying stress).

Make the Detox Salad

In a bowl, toss cucumber and tomatoes with sumac, salt, and pepper. Set aside.

Assemble the Bowls

1. Spoon golden rice into bowls. Top with charred chicken, fresh salad, and a dollop of tzatziki.
2. Finish with chopped parsley. Serve with flatbread if desired—and extra tzatziki because joy matters too.

CHARLENE'S CAULIFLOWER "MASHED POTATOES" WITH SPRING ONIONS

Recipe by Charlene Bollinger, Co-Founder of The Truth About Cancer.

Total time: 30 minutes
Serves: 4–5

Ingredients:

2 heads of cauliflower
6 tablespoons ghee (or grass-fed butter)
1 clove garlic, minced
1½ green onions, minced
¼ cup Greek yogurt (grass-fed)
¼ cup cheddar cheese (grass-fed)
½ teaspoon sea salt
⅛ teaspoon pepper

Instructions:

1. Remove the outer leaves and chop two heads of cauliflower down to the florets.
2. Place the cauliflower into a medium pan with about two inches of water and cover with a lid. Steam the cauliflower until fully cooked and tender, then set aside.
3. Add five tablespoons of the ghee, one clove minced garlic, and one chopped green onion to a medium saucepan over medium heat. Sauté for 5 minutes or until soft.
4. Add the steamed cauliflower to a large bowl with the sautéed garlic and green onions, greek yogurt, ¼ cup of the grated cheddar cheese, salt, and pepper. Whip together with an electric hand mixer until smooth.
5. Place your smooth mashed cauliflower mixture in a large bowl and garnish with half of a chopped green onion and the one extra

tablespoon of chopped green onion and the one extra tablespoon of melted ghee on top. Serve warm.

Notes: You can also use a food processor to smooth the ingredients together, instead of an electric hand mixer, or mash and mix thoroughly by hand.

RECIPE WITH BEEF TALLOW

Ways to Use Beef Tallow

Tallow has a rich, savory flavor that enhances various dishes, from roasting and frying to searing. Use it to make French fries, onion rings, fried chicken, and golden-brown vegetables. It is terrific for searing meat. It helps you create a crispy crust that keeps the meat juicy and flavorful. Use it for roasting vegetables like brussels sprouts and potatoes; it gives them a caramelized texture. Melt the tallow, then toss in the veggies and roast until golden brown. Add broth and flour for a rich, flavorful gravy or sauce. It also lends flavor to pastries, biscuits, and piecrust.

CHERIE'S OLD-FASHIONED BEEF TALLOW CORNBREAD

Total time: 30–35 minutes
Serves 6–8

Ingredients:

- 1 cup fine organic cornmeal
- 1 cup all-purpose, unbleached organic flour or gluten-free flour such as garbanzo bean flour
- 1 tablespoon baking powder
- 1 teaspoon sea salt
- 2 large pastured eggs
- 1 cup pastured buttermilk
- ¼ cup + 1 tablespoon melted beef tallow, divided
- 2 tablespoons honey, pure maple syrup, or coconut nectar

Instructions:

1. Preheat the oven to 400°F. Set aside a 9-inch cast-iron skillet.
2. Stir together the cornmeal, flour, baking powder, and salt in a large bowl.
3. In another bowl, beat the eggs until frothy, then stir in the buttermilk, melted beef tallow, and sweetener.

4. Pour the wet ingredients into the dry ingredients and mix until just combined—being careful not to overmix! (Lumps are okay and prevent tough cornbread.)
5. Place the empty cast-iron skillet in the preheated oven for 5 minutes to heat it.
6. Remove the hot skillet from the oven and add 1 tablespoon of additional beef tallow to coat the bottom and sides.
7. Immediately pour the batter into the hot skillet. It should sizzle. (Tip: The hot skillet gives you that country-style crispy crust.)
8. Bake at 400°F for 20 to 25 minutes or until the top is golden brown and a toothpick inserted in the center comes out clean.
9. Let the cornbread cool in the skillet for 10 minutes before slicing. (Resting helps the cornbread set perfectly.)

Liana's recipes are from her books *Cancer-Free with Food, The Earth Diet, 10-Minute Recipes,* and *Anxiety-Free with Food.*

Cherie's recipes are from her books *The Anti-Inflammation Diet, Souping is the New Juicing, The Coconut Diet,* and *Sugar Knockout.*

CHAPTER 5

The Good Fats and Oils Shopping Guide and Resources

When choosing oils and fats, prioritize quality, organic, freshness, sourcing, and authenticity. Select cold-pressed or expeller-pressed oils to preserve nutrients and avoid toxic by-products created by chemical extraction and high heat. Choose extra-virgin olive oil or avocado oil in dark glass bottles to reduce oxidation, and always check for a harvest date or best-by date. Buy nut oils in small quantities, refrigerate after opening, and seal tightly, because they spoil quickly. For traditional fats like butter or beef tallow, choose grass-fed and pasture-raised for better nutrition, including omega-3 fatty acids, CLA, and vitamin K2. Pasture-raised means the cows are roaming free in the pasture, eating grass, as they should be. Avoid heavily refined or hydrogenated products, and avoid oils in plastic bottles due to microplastics. The best fats are always those closest to their natural state.

Tips in a Nutshell

- Buy extra-virgin over virgin.
- When buying nut oils, refrigerate after opening and seal tightly to prevent oxidation.
- Choose cold-pressed over expeller-pressed (cold-pressed uses no or minimal heat, 122 °F or below; expeller-pressed uses some heat but no chemicals).
- Avoid all oils extracted with chemicals.

- Choose oils in dark bottles to protect from light and oxidation.
- For the most nutritious oil, choose cold-pressed, unrefined oil.

Virgin and Extra-Virgin Oil

The terms "virgin" and "extra-virgin" indicate how the oil was processed and its quality.

Extra-Virgin: Highest quality. First cold-pressing with no heat or chemicals; low acidity; maximum flavor, nutrients, and antioxidants; purest and most unrefined.
Virgin: Cold-pressed and unrefined, but slightly higher acidity and milder flavor than extra virgin.

In short: extra-virgin = top tier; virgin = still high quality, but slightly lower in taste and purity.

The Amazing Oils for Your Kitchen

Almond Oil

Choose only cold-pressed almond oil with no added ingredients (fragrances, parabens, sulfates). Buy in dark bottles and refrigerate after opening. Great for baking, desserts, and plant-based butter and cheeses.

Avocado Oil

Made by pressing/centrifuging avocado flesh; some brands refine it, while unrefined preserves more nutrients. Because avocado oil is prone to fraud, sourcing matters: UC Davis researchers found that 82 percent of samples tested were stale before the expiration date or mixed with other oils.[1]

For a reputable brand, check out Primal Kitchen (founded by Mark Sisson), including pure avocado oil and their Air Fryer Oil made of avocado and MCT coconut oil, plus avocado-oil salad dressings.

Coconut Oil

Virgin coconut oil (VCO) is extracted from fresh coconut meat and offers MCTs and antioxidants. (There is no distinction between extra-virgin and virgin coconut oil. Extra-virgin in this case is just a marketing tool.) Refined coconut oil has a higher smoke point (~450°F) and a neutral taste, though with fewer nutrients. Organic indicates it is grown without pesticides.

For a reputable brand, check out Dr. Bronner's Organic Virgin Coconut Oil.

Flaxseed Oil

Cold-pressed flaxseed oil is rich in omega-3s (ALA). Do not cook with it. Refrigerate, use only in cold applications, and discard after 6 months if not used. Use on salads or in smoothies, or drizzle over soups and bone broths before serving. You can also take 1 to 2 teaspoons before bed to support omega-3 intake and brain function. Liana discusses flax oil's role in cancer prevention and healing in *Cancer Free with Food*. For a reputable brand, check out Barleans.

Hempseed Oil

Only purchase cold-pressed (avoid solvent-extracted). Rich in omega-3s, including GLA; arginine supports cardiovascular health. Do not cook with it. Best for smoothies, raw desserts, and cold dishes, or drizzled over hot food.

Macadamia Nut Oil

Cold-pressed or expeller-pressed. Look for clarity, golden-yellow color, and mild aroma. Naturally high smoke point (400°F–450°F), making it ideal for high-heat cooking. Great for searing, roasting, baking, dressings, mayo, and aioli.

MCT Oil

Choose organic coconut-sourced MCT oil (not palm), ideally C8 or C8/C10, solvent-free and hexane-free, with clean sourcing and no fillers. Dark glass is best. Add to coffee for steadier energy and fewer jitters; add to smoothies for brain and nervous system fuel. In *Cancer-Free with Food*, Liana includes MCT oil in the Chemo Brain Smoothie because ketones provide an alternative fuel source for the brain.

Olive Oil

Look for extra-virgin, harvest date (most recent fall/spring), best-by date, certification seals, and single-country origin. Avoid oils labeled "pure" or "light." Olive oil is frequently adulterated; reports and investigations have documented widespread counterfeiting and mislabeling.[2]

Use these guidelines:

1. "Extra-virgin" on the label
2. Forest green or deep yellow-green color
3. Peppery taste and fruity aroma
4. Prefer California oils meeting strict standards (when applicable)
5. For reputable brands, check out Primal Kitchen Extra Virgin Olive Oil (Spain and Tunisia) and Kosterina Organic Extra Virgin Olive Oil (Greece).

Omega-3 Oils

Omega-3s (DHA/EPA) support the brain, nervous system, inflammation balance, and cellular repair, especially in a modern diet skewed toward omega-6 fats.

For a trusted brand, check out Global Healing Omega-3 Fatty Acids (liquid formula for absorption). Use code Liana for 10 percent off at GlobalHealing.com.

Pumpkin Seed Oil

Cold-pressed, dark green/deep red, nutty flavor. Use in dressings, smoothies, finishing, desserts; not for cooking. Research notes hair-growth benefits and men's urinary/BPH support.[3, 4] Parasites hate pumpkin seeds, so use often.

Sesame Seed Oil

Cold-pressed from raw or toasted seeds (toasted has lower smoke point). Used for sautéing, stir-frying, finishing, and dressings. Helps lower blood pressure and inflammation.

Walnut Oil

Cold-pressed; not for cooking. Use for drizzling, dressings, and sauces. Supports heart and brain health and improves lipid profiles; rich in omega-3s.

Nourishing Animal Fats

Beef Tallow

Choose grass-fed, pasture-raised tallow with minimal processing and no additives. Prefer suet-derived for cooking. Grass-fed tallow is typically deeper yellow due to beta -carotene and contains more CLA and omega-3s.

Grass-Fed Butter

Choose real grass-fed cultured butter: "Real cultured butter is crafted by adding live bacterial cultures to the cream before churning, similar to preparing yogurt."[5] Look for "live active cultures" or "cultured cream." If you see "lactic acid," it's usually a shortcut. Kerrygold unsalted is cultured; salted is not. Grass-fed butter offers better CLA and omega-3 balance, plus vitamin K2 and beta-carotene[6]

Avoid spreads/blends and tub "butters"—they often contain seed oils.

Fun Fact: Butter is an ancient food and mentioned in the Old Testament ten times, the first in Genesis when Abraham serves butter along with milk and meat to his guests, showing it is a wholesome, desirable food.

For a reputable brand, check out Truly Butter or Vital Farms.

If you're in Utah, visit Redmond Heritage Farm stores for raw butter (and raw milk); they may offer online ordering soon.

Ghee

Choose ghee from grass-fed, pasture-raised cows, with no additives. It should be clear and golden with no cloudiness or sediment. Ghee is clarified butter: lactose- and casein-free, higher smoke point, shelf-stable, and nutty in flavor.

Healthy Fats = Happy Body

Choosing the right oils and fats isn't just about labels—it's about clarity over marketing. The fats you buy shape your meals, your metabolism, and your vitality. Big money has influenced the fats and oils market—but change happens when people stop buying the products that made them sick. Spread the word.

Resources That Help You Shop Wisely and Eat Out with Direction

For the brands we have vetted, recommend, and trust, and a free downloadable shopping guide, go to thetruthabouotseedoils.com.

Seed Oil Scout (www.SeedOilScout.com)

Get the Seed Oil Scout app; it is a community-driven map of restaurant ingredients and sourcing. Wherever you are in the United States, you can type in your location and find restaurants near you that are seed oil–free. Find restaurants using natural fats like beef tallow and avocado oil and organic produce.

The Templeton List (TempletonList.com)

Your guide to the healthiest restaurants in America. This is a list of restaurants that use only healthy ingredients like organic. You can search for thousands of hand-picked restaurants, featuring fresh, healthy food you can feel good about eating.

Wake Up and Read the Labels by Jen Smiley

A helpful app designed to decode food labels while you shop. Read the Labels highlights ingredients such as seed oils, additives, and preservatives, and guides users toward cleaner swaps, without overwhelm. It's designed to give people clarity and confidence when choosing food. Unlike most apps, it specifically flags seed oils, such as sunflower oil.

Find it at www.jensmiley.com.

WAPF Shopping Guide

This is the Weston A. Price Foundation guide to healthy shopping, which lists companies and farms that prioritize the highest-quality and most nutrient-dense foods. Find it at https://www.westonaprice.org/digital-journal/shopping-guide-2022/#gsc.tab=0.

Copow Foods

Copow Foods is a great resource for anyone wanting seed-oil-free convenience without compromising on taste. They offer pre-made, regenerative organic high-protein meals made with real ingredients like pasture-raised steak, wild-caught fish, organic chicken, vegetables, and sweet potatoes—all low sugar, low carb, and deeply satisfying. Cowpow also operates as a seed-oil-free convenience store, where you can shop for snacks, protein bars, olive oil, and everyday grocery staples, all carefully curated with no seed oils. Use code seedoilfree at checkout for a discount.

Environmental Working Group (EWG.org)

Download the app for the Dirty Dozen (the most heavily sprayed with pesticides) and the Clean Fifteen.

Ways to Connect with Liana Werner-Gray

TheEarthDiet.com is Liana's website where you can find free recipes, healing protocols and a free 3-Day Cleanse. Connect with Liana on social media @LianaWernerGray and @TheEarthDiet across all platforms. Additionally, you can find Liana's books *The Earth Diet*, *10-Minute Recipes*, *Anxiety-Free with Food*, and *Cancer-Free with Food* on Amazon and in bookstores globally.

Ways to Connect with Cherie Calbom

Visit juiceladyinfo.com or juiceladycherie.com for information on juicing, nutrition, and a healthy lifestyle with a variety of online programs and Raw Food Retreats. For a discount on Cherie's favorite juicer, the Nama J2, use code Juicelady. Sign up for Cherie's Newsletter for recipes and nutrition tips. Schedule a nutrition consultation with Cherie: cherie@juicladycherie.com. You can also find Cherie's books, including *Juicing for Life*, *The Big Book of Juices and Green Smoothies*, and *The Anti-Inflammation Diet*, on Amazon and in bookstores globally. Connect with Cherie on IG @JuiceLadyCherie and Facebook @TheJuiceLady.

About the Authors

Liana Werner-Gray, CN, is a functional nutritionist and the bestselling author of four books, including *The Earth Diet* and *Cancer Free with Food*, one of the top one hundred cancer books of all time. She is a sixteen-year cancer survivor and has been deeply committed to educating people on prevention and healing through natural nutrition since 2009. Liana is a regular personality on TV, including *Good Day NY*, Fox News, and KTLA LA News.

Cherie Calbom, MS, celebrated worldwide as "The Juice Lady," is a trailblazer in whole-food nutrition and the juicing revolution. With an MS in nutrition and a passion for transforming health through fresh, vibrant foods, she has authored thirty-six books that have collectively sold over 3.5 million copies. Her global bestseller *Juicing for Life* has empowered 2 million readers to reclaim vitality. From serving as George Foreman's nutritionist to advising the Royal Family of the UAE, Cherie's influence spans continents and cultures. Her mother died of breast cancer when she was six years old, creating a passionate desire to help people heal and prevent disease. A dynamic voice in wellness, Cherie has been featured on Fox News, NBC, CBS, ABC, CNN, CBN, TBN, and *It's Supernatural*, inspiring millions with her message: Health is not just a goal; it's a lifestyle.

Acknowledgments

We would like to extend our deepest gratitude to Robert F. Kennedy Jr., a true hero, for helping create a platform where truth can finally be heard. Because of your courage and leadership, millions of people are now aware of what seed oils are and why they matter. You have given this movement a voice when it was most needed.

Thank you to Tony Lyons, CEO of MAHA Action and Skyhorse Publishing, for your tireless work, integrity, and unwavering commitment to publishing truth in a world that often resists it.

Thank you to the Skyhorse Publishing team for everything you do; you are changing the world one book at a time.

Thank you to Daniela Rapp for her dedication and work behind the scenes, and to Cherie for encouraging this book into existence.

We would also like to thank Dr. Cate Shanahan, one of the leading pioneers in exposing the truth about seed oils. Your groundbreaking work, especially the creation of The Hateful Eight, has helped awaken the world to the profound impact industrial oils have on our health and food system.

Thank you, Joe Polish, for connecting so many dots, as you always do, and helping this work come together.

Thank you to everyone who contributed recipes to this book: Cheryl Hines, Marla Maples, Vani Hari, Dr Josh Axe, Jordan Rubin, Dr Austin Lake, Dr Will Cole, Dr Jess Peatross, Ann Louise Gittleman, Chef Pete Evans, Kelly Ryerson, Suzi Griswold, Maria Marlowe, Leah Wilson and her momma Mandy, Charlene Bollinger, and Lexi Noel.

Endnotes

Chapter 1: Liquid Lies: The Seed Oil Scandal

1 Cherie Calbom, *The Coconut Diet: The Secret Ingredient That Helps You Lose Weight While You Eat Your Favorite Foods* (New York: Time Warner, 2005).

2 Nina Teicholz, *The Big Fat Surprise: Why Butter, Meat and Cheese Belong in a Healthy Diet* (New York: Simon & Schuster, 2014, 3–4).

3 Martha N. Gardner and Allan M. Brandt. "The Doctors' Choice Is America's Choice": The Physician in US Cigarette Advertisements, 1930–1953." *Am J Public Health*. 96, no. 2 (February 2006): 222–32. doi: 10.2105/AJPH.2005.066654.

4 Frank B. Hu, Meir J. Stampfer, Eric B. Rimm et al. "A Prospective Study of Egg Consumption and Risk of Cardiovascular Disease in Men and Women." *JAMA*.

5 Teicholz, 3–4.

6 Jason Andrade, Aneez Mohamed, Jiri Frohlich, Andrew Ignaszewski. "Ancel Keys and the Lipid Hypothesis." *BCMJ* 51, no. 2 (March 2009): 66–72.

7 "Ansel Keys Study: A Closer Look." Herstel Health. https://herstelhealth.com/2025/01/ansel-keys-study-a-closer-look/.

8 Joseph Tiscani, "How Procter & Gamble Paid to Shape America's Diet: Lessons from a Lard War. "https://www.linkedin.com/pulse/how-procter-gamble-paid-shape-americas-diet-lessons-woxwc/.

9 "Eric Decker Discusses Seed Oils with Media." UMass Amherst. https://www.umass.edu/natural-sciences/news/eric-decker-seed-oils.

10 Caitlin Dow. "Seed Oils: Are They Healthy or Harmful?" https://www.cspi.org/article/seed-oils-are-they-healthy-or-harmful.

11 "Hexane."EPAHazardSummary.https://www.epa.gov/sites/default/files/2016-09/documents/hexane.pdf.

Chapter 2: Seed Oils Cause Anxiety, Depression, Alzheimer's, Dementia, and Worse

1 McKenzie Beard. "Bolivian Community with Just 1% Dementia and the 'Healthiest Hearts in the World' Follow This Diet." *New York Post*. https://nypost.com/2025/02/25/bolivian-communitys-diet-linked-to-heart-health-no-dementia/.

2 Jenette Restivo. "Guide to the Mediterranean Diet." *Harvard Health*. https://www.health.harvard.edu/staying-healthy/guide-to-the-mediterranean-diet.

3 "Adventist Health Studies." Wikipedia. https://en.wikipedia.org/wiki/Adventist_Health_Studies.

4 "European Prospective Investigation into Cancer and Nutrition." Wikipedia. https://en.wikipedia.org/wiki/European_Prospective_Investigation_into_Cancer_and_Nutritio.

5 Muhammad Sohail Khan. "Type 2 Diabetes and Alzheimer's Disease: Molecular Mechanisms and Therapeutic Insights with a Focus on Anthocyanin." *Journal of Dementia and Alzheimer's Disease* 3, no. 1 (January 15, 2026): 5. https://doi.org/10.3390/jdad3010005.

6 Francisco Moreno et al. "Influence of the Degree of Unsaturation in Fish Oil Supplements on Oxidative Stress and Protein Carbonylation in the Cerebral Cortex and Cerebellum of Healthy Rats." *Antioxidants (Basel)* 13, no. 11 (November 17, 2024): 13. https://pmc.ncbi.nlm.nih.gov/articles/PMC11591239/.

7 Dong D. Wang. "Association of Specific Dietary Fats With Total and Cause-Specific Mortality." *JAMA Internal Medicine* 176, no. 8.

8 Giulia Crouch. "RFK Jr. Says They Are Poisoning Us, Influencers Call Them Unnatural—but What Is the Truth About Seed Oils?" *The Guardian* (March 29, 2025). https://www.theguardian.com/science/2025/mar/29/rfk-jr-says-they-are-poisoning-us-influencers-call-them-unnatural-but-what-is-the-truth-about-seed-oils.

9 "Heart Surgeon Speaks Out on What Really Causes Heart Disease." https://people.uncw.edu/imperialm/UNCW/PLS_506/242516-Heart-Surgeon-Speaks-Out-On-What-Really-Causes-Heart-Disease.pdf.

10 Martin Loef et al. "The Omega-6/Omega-3 Ratio and Dementia or Cognitive Decline: A Systematic Review on Human Studies and Biological Evidence." J Nutr *Gerontol Geriatr* 32, no. 1 (2013): 1–23.

11 Nina Teicholz. "The Big Fat Surprise: Toxic Heated Oils." Weston A. Price Foundation. https://www.westonaprice.org/health-topics/know-your-fats/the-big-fat-surprise-toxic-heated-oils/#gsc.tab=0.

12 "Is Sunflower Oil Inflammatory?" *Biology Insights*. https://biologyinsights.com/is-sunflower-oil-inflammatory/#:~:text=Once%20consumed%2C%20linoleic%20acid%20is%20metabolized%20into%20arachidonic,by%20enzymes%20like%20cyclooxygenase%20%28COX%29%20and%20lipoxygenase%20%28LOX%29.

13 Amir Y. Taha. "Linoleic Acid—Good or Bad for the Brain?" npj science of food 4 (2020). https://www.nature.com/articles/s41538-019-0061-9.

14 Godefroid Charbon, Matthew T. Cabeen, and Christine Jacobs-Walter. "Bacterial Intermediate Filaments: In Vivo Assembly, Organization, and Dynamics of Crescentin." *Genes Dev.* 1, no. 23 (May 2009): 1131–44.

15 Wenqiang Fang. "Neuroinflammation: Mechanisms, Dual Roles, and Therapeutic Strategies in Neurological Disorders." *Mol Biol.* 47, no. 6 (June 4, 2025).

16 Xin Deng et al. "Corrigendum: HAX-1 Protects Glioblastoma Cells from Apoptosis Through the Akt1 Pathway." *Cell. Neurosci.* 13 (January 30, 2019).

17 Corinne Joffre. "n-3 Polyunsaturated Fatty Acids and Their Derivates Reduce Neuroinflammation During Aging." *Nutrients* 12, no. 3 (February 27, 2020): 647.

18 Nicole E. Spruijt et al. "A Systematic Review of Randomized Controlled Trials Exploring the Effect of Immunomodulative Interventions on Infection, Organ Failure, and Mortality in Trauma Patients." *Crit Care* 14, no. 4 (2010).

19 Jens-Michael Jensen et al. "Disseminated Porokeratosis Palmaris and Plantaris Treated with Imiquimod Cream to Prevent Malignancy." *PMD* 85, no. 6 (2005).

20 Volkan Karataşlı et al. "Clinicopathologic Evaluation of Uterine Smooth Muscle Tumors of Uncertain Malignant Potential (STUMP): A Single Center Experience." *J Gynecol Obstet Hum Reprod.* 48, no. 8 (October 2019).

21 F. Dumas et al. "Chromosome Painting of the Pygmy Tree Shrew Shows That No Derived Cytogenetic Traits Link Primates and Scandentia." *Cytogenet Genome Res* 136, no. 3 (2012): 175–79.

22 Jian Duan et al. "Effects of Rainfall Patterns and Land Cover on the Subsurface Flow Generation of Sloping Ferralsols in Southern China." *PLoS One* 12, no. 8 (August 8, 2017).

23 "Imbalanced Omega 6 to Omega-3 Ratios Linked to Chronic Diseases." *Mental Health Daily.* https://mentalhealthdaily.com/2023/10/31/imbalanced-omega-6-omega-3-ratios-chronic-diseases/.

24 "Heart Surgeon Speaks Out on What Really Causes Heart Disease."

25 Stefan Broselid. "Dietary Omega-3/6 Balance: New Research Links Fatty Acid Ratios to Chronic Disease and Longevity." https://ecs.education/2025/03/12/omega-balance-inflammation-longevity/.

26 "Omega-6 Fatty Acid Promotes the Growth of an Aggressive Type of Breast Cancer." Weill Cornell Medicine. https://meyercancer.weill.cornell.edu/news/2025-04-01/omega-6-fatty-acid-promotes-growth-aggressive-type-breast-cancer.

27 "Cooking Vegetable Oil Releases Toxic Chemicals Linked to Cancer" https://www.foodmatters.com/article/cooking-vegetable-oil-releases-toxic-chemicals-linked-to-cancer.

28 Loef et al.

29 Jennifer Prince. "Omega-6 Fatty Acids May Increase Fat Accumulation, Insulin Resistance in Subjects with Type 2 Diabetes, Study Suggests." *Nutritional Outlook.* https://www.nutritionaloutlook.com/view/omega-6-fatty-acids-may-increase-fat-accumulation-insulin-resistance-subjects-type-2-diabetes-study#:~:text=The%20researchers%20found%20that%20a%20high%20serum%20dihomo-%CE%B3-.linolenic,resistance%20in%20Japanese%20subjects%20with%20type%202%20diabetes.

30 "Heart Surgeon Speaks Out on What Really Causes Heart Disease."

31 Mohammadi et al., "Linoleic Acid Intake and Psychological Disorders." *Frontiers in Nutrition, Nutritional Epidemiology* 9 (2022) https://www.frontiersin.org/journals/nutrition/articles/10.3389/fnut.2022.841282/full.

32 Nathan Gray. "Study Links Trans Fat Intake to Depression." *Food Navigator.* https://www.foodnavigator.com/Article/2011/02/02/Study-links-trans-fat-intake-to-depression/.

33 Mohammadi et al.
34 Jenna Birch. "Unprocessed vs. Processed Foods: Key Differences." Health.com. https://www.health.com/nutrition/eat-clean-give-up-processed-foods.
35 "Omega-6 Fatty Acid Promotes the Growth of an Aggressive Type of Breast Cancer."
36 "Omega-6 Fatty Acid Promotes the Growth of an Aggressive Type of Breast Cancer."
37 Lauren J. Young. "Ultraprocessed Foods High in Seed Oils Could Be Fueling Colon Cancer Risk." *Scientific American* (December 13, 2024).
38 Ah Young Lee et al. "Effects of Vegetable Oils with Different Fatty Acid Compositions on Cognition and Memory Ability in Aβ25-35-Induced Alzheimer's Disease Mouse Model." *J Med Food* 19, no. 10 (October 2016): 912–921. https://pubmed.ncbi.nlm.nih.gov/27696934/.
39 Ian Sample. "Women with Alzheimer's Have Unusually Low Omega Fatty Acid Levels, Study Finds." *The Guardian* (August 20, 2025). https://www.theguardian.com/science/2025/aug/20/women-with-alzheimers-have-unusually-low-omega-fatty-acid-levels-study-finds.
40 "MICOIL Study in Greece Finds That a Diet Rich in Early Harvest Extra Virgin Olive Oil May Help Protect Against Cognitive Impairment." *Alzheimer Europe*. https://www.alzheimer-europe.org/news/micoil-study-greece-finds-diet-rich-early-harvest-extra-virgin-olive-oil-may-help-protect?language=en&language_content_entity=en&utm_source=chatgpt.com.
41 Heidi Godman. "Harvard Study: High Olive Oil Consumption Associated with Longevity." *Harvard Health*. https://www.health.harvard.edu/staying-healthy/harvard-study-high-olive-oil-consumption-associated-with-longevity.
42 Cecile A. Obeid et al. "Adherence to the Mediterranean Diet Among Adults in Mediterranean Countries: A Systematic Literature Review." *European Journal of Nutrition* 61 (April 22, 2022): 3327–44. https://link.springer.com/article/10.1007/s00394-022-02885-0.
43 Loef et al.
44 Gori Pooja et al. "Oxidative Stress and Free Radicals in Disease Pathogenesis: A Review." *Discover Medicine* 2 (April 14, 2025). https://link.springer.com/article/10.1007/s44337-025-00303-y.
45 "'Good Fats' and Inflammation: More Complex than First Thought." University of Queensland. https://news.uq.edu.au/2025-06-30-good-fats-and-inflammation-more-complex-first-thought.
46 "How Inflammation Affects Hair Follicles: Unraveling the Science Behind Hair Loss." *Arthritis Care of Texas*. https://aoccb.com/how-inflammation-affects-hair-follicles-unraveling-the-science-behind-hair-loss/.
47 Ah-Rang Choi. "Antagonistic Activities and Probiotic Potential of Lactic Acid Bacteria Derived From a Plant-Based Fermented Food." *Sec. Food Microbiology* 9 (2018). https://www.frontiersin.org/journals/microbiology/articles/10.3389/fmicb.2018.01963/full.
48 Amro M. Soliman et al. "Acute Inflammation in Tissue Healing." *International Journal of Molecular Sciences* 24, no. 1 (December 29, 2022).

49 D. Preston et al. "Ecological Consequences of Parasitism." *Nature Education Knowledge* 3, no. 10 (2010): 47.

50 Pallee Shree et al. "Biofilms: Understanding the Structure and Contribution Towards Bacterial Resistance in Antibiotics." *Medicine in Microecology* 16 (June 2023). https://www.sciencedirect.com/science/article/pii/S2590097823000095.

51 São Paulo Research Foundation. "Diabetes Breakthrough: Fish Oil May Reverse Insulin Resistance." *SciTechDaily*. https://scitechdaily.com/diabetes-breakthrough-fish-oil-may-reverse-insulin-resistance/.

52 James J. DiNicolantonio. "Importance of Maintaining a Low Omega–6/Omega–3 Ratio for Reducing Inflammation." *BMJ* 5, no. 2 (November 26, 2018).

53 Jacqueline K. Innes. "Omega-6 Fatty Acids and Inflammation." Review Prostaglandins Leukot Essent Fatty Acids 132 (May 2018): 41–48.

54 "Heart Surgeon Speaks Out on What Really Causes Heart Disease."

55 Harold E. Bays. "Adoposopathy: Is "Sick Fat" a Cardiovascular Disease?" *J Am Coll Cardiol* 21, no. 25 (June 2011): 2461–73.

56 Wayne Eskridge. "The Seed Oil Debate Is Ramping Up, What You Need to Know About Omega 6 Oils." Fatty Liver Foundation (March 24, 2025). https://www.fattyliverfoundation.org/what_you_need_to_know_about_omega_6_oils.

57 Napapan Kangwan. "Perilla Seed Oil Alleviates Gut Dysbiosis, Intestinal Inflammation and Metabolic Disturbance in Obese-Insulin-Resistant Rats." *Nutrients* 13, no. 9 (September 8, 2021).

58 H. Duve. "Callatostatins: Neuropeptides from the Blowfly Calliphora vomitoria with Sequence Homology to Cockroach Allatostatins." *Comparative Study Proc Natl Acad Sci* 90, no. 6 (March 15, 1993): 2456–60.

59 "Linoleic Acid, Mitochondria, Gut Microbiome, and Metabolic Health: A Mechanistic Review." https://media.mercola.com/PDF/research-papers/linoleic-acid-mitochondria-gut-microbiome-and-metabolic-health-simplified.pdf.

60 Tyler Ransom and Tucker Goodrich. "Are Vegetable Seed Oils Fueling the Obesity Epidemic?" https://tyleransom.github.io/research/obesity-seed-oils.pdf.

61 J. R. Hibbeln, L. R. Nieminen, W. E. Lands et al. "Increasing Homicide Rates and Linoleic Acid Consumption Among Five Western Countries, 1961–2000." *Lipids* (2004). Full text abstract: https://pubmed.ncbi.nlm.nih.gov/15736917/.

62 Mark Hyman, MD. "Are Seed Oils Bad for You? Here's What You Need to Know." https://drhyman.com/blogs/content/are-seed-oils-bad-for-you-here-s-what-you-need-to-know/.

Chapter 3: Everything You Need to Know About Oils and Fats

1 "List of Fatty Acids." Tuscany Diet. https://www.tuscany-diet.net/lipids/list-of-fatty-acids/#google_vignette.

2 C. C. Akoh and D. B. Min. *Food Lipids: Chemistry, Nutrition, and Biotechnology,* 3rd ed. (CRC Press, 2008).

3 Ching K. Chow. Fatty Acids in *Foods and Their Health Implications,* 3rd ed. (Routledge, 2008).

4 Dr. Eric Berg. "Understanding Cholesterol Levels and Numbers." https://www.drberg.com/blog/how-to-read-and-understand-cholesterol-numbers.

5 Cate Shanahan, MD. *Deep Nutrition* (New York: Flatiron Books 2018).

6 Mark Hünlich, Kelly J. Begin, Joseph A. Gorga, David E. Fishbaugher, Martin M. LeWinter, and Peter VanBuren. "Protein Kinase A Mediated Modulation of Acto-myosin Kinetics." *J Mol Cell Cardiol* 38 (January 2005). https://pubmed.ncbi.nlm.nih.gov/15623428/ and https://pubmed.ncbi.nlm.nih.gov/26747615/.

7 James E. Dalen et al. "The Epidemic of the 20th Century: Coronary Heart Disease." *Am J Med* 127, no. 9 (September 2014). https://pubmed.ncbi.nlm.nih.gov/24811552/.

8 H. Kaunitz. "Medium Chain Triglycerides (MCT) in Aging and Arteriosclerosis." *J Environ Pathol Toxicol Oncol* (1986).

9 Maria Luz Fernandez and Ana Gabriela Murillo. "Is There a Correlation Between Dietary and Blood Cholesterol? Evidence from Epidemiological Data and Clinical Interventions." *Nutrients* 14, no. 10 (May 23, 2022). https://pmc.ncbi.nlm.nih.gov/articles/PMC9143438/.

10 Bruce Fife. *The Healing Miracles of Coconut Oil* (London:: Piccadilly Books, 2003), 26–32.

11 Fife, 27.

12 Mary Enig. "Coconut: In Support of Good Health in the 21st Century." https://www.coconutoil.co.nz/PDF/Coconut_Good_Health_21st_Century.pdf.

13 Enig.

14 Fife, 28.

15 Artemis P. Simopoulos. "The Importance of the Omega-6/Omega-3 Fatty Acid Ratio in Cardiovascular Disease and Other Chronic Diseases." *SEBM* 233, no. 6 (2008). https://journals.sagepub.com/doi/10.3181/0711-MR-311; https://pmc.ncbi.nlm.nih.gov/articles/PMC7037798/.

16 "22 Foods High in Trans Fat You Should Avoid." *New Health Advisor.* https://www.newhealthadvisor.org/Foods-High-in-Trans-Fat.html?utm.

17 Shekari S, Fathi S, Roumi Z, et al. "Association between dietary intake of fatty acids and colorectal cancer, a case-control study." *Front Nutr.* 2022;9:856408. https://pmc.ncbi.nlm.nih.gov/articles/PMC9576465/.

18 "Why Does Olive Oil Keep Heart Attack and Stroke at Bay?" *Medical News Today.* https://www.medicalnewstoday.com/articles/323007).

19 Heidi Godman. "Harvard Study: High Olive Oil Consumption Associated with Longevity." *Harvard Health* (April 1, 2022). https://www.health.harvard.edu/staying-healthy/harvard-study-high-olive-oil-consumption-associated-with-longevity/.

20 John Richardson. "The Science Behind Extra Virgin Olive Oil's Health Benefits." *ASB.* https://asb.org.uk/blog/02/2025/the-science-behind-extra-virgin-olive-oils-health-benefits/8428/.

21 Orla M. Finucane et al. "Monounsaturated Fatty Acid–Enriched High-Fat Diets Impede Adipose NLRP3 Inflammasome-Mediated IL-1β Secretion and Insulin Resistance Despite Obesity." *Obesity Studies* 64, no. 6 (June 2015). https://diabetesjournals.org/diabetes/article-abstract/64/6/2116/34911/.

22 S. K. Yeap et al., 2015. Antistress and antioxidant effects of virgin coconut oil in vivo. Experimental and Therapeutic Medicine – Jan 2015; 9(1): 39–42.

23 Lindsey Shapiro. "Coconut Oil and Green Tea Lead to Gait, Balance Gains in MS Patients." https://multiplesclerosisnewstoday.com/news-posts/2023/02/02/coconut-oil-green-tea-supplements-lead-ms-balance-gait-gains-study/.

24 M. D. White et al. "Enhanced Postprandial Energy Expenditure with Medium-Chain Fatty Acid Feeding Is Attenuated After 14 d in Premenopausal Women." *American Journal of Clinical Nutrition* (1999).

25 "Evidence-Based Health Benefits of Avocado Oil." https://www.healthline.com/nutrition/9-avocado-oil-benefits#heart-health.

26 David Calderón Guzmán et al. "Oleic Acid Protects Against Oxidative Stress Exacerbated by Cytarabine and Doxorubicin in Rat Brain." *Anticancer Agents Med Chem* 16, no. 11 (2016): 1491–95. https://pubmed.ncbi.nlm.nih.gov/27141883/.

27 John Staughton. "8 Surprising Macadamia Nut Oil Benefits." *Organic Facts* (April 15, 2024). https://www.organicfacts.net/health-benefits/oils/macadamia-nut-oil.html.

28 Dianne A. Hyson. "Almonds and Almond Oil Have Similar Effects on Plasma Lipids and LDL Oxidation in Healthy Men and Women." *Journal of Nutrition* 132, no. 4 (April 2002): 703–7. https://jn.nutrition.org/article/S0022-3166(22)15035-2/fulltext.

29 Hala Gali-Muhtasib et al. "Thymoquinone Extracted from Black Seed Triggers Apoptotic Cell Death in Human Colorectal Cancer Cells via a p53-Dependent Mechanism." *Int J Oncol* 24, no. 4 (October 2004): 857–66.

30 Sophie Dubois. "Black Seed Oil and Parasites: Evidence-Based Analysis." https://spice.alibaba.com/spice-basics/does-black-seed-oil-kill-parasites.

31 Liya Denney, et al. "Food Sources of Energy and Nutrients in Infants, Toddlers, and Young Children." Mexican National Health and Nutrition Survey 2012. *Nutrients.* 2017 May 13;9(5):494. doi: 10.3390/nu9050494.

32 Hana Duranova et. al. "Coconut-sourced MCT oil: its potential health benefits beyond traditionacoconut oil." *Phytochemistry Reviews*, May 2, 2024 Volume 24, pages 659–700, (2025).

33 "Pumpkin Seed Oil: Is It Good for You?" https://www.webmd.com/diet/pumpkin-seed-oil-good-for-you.

34 Ruzena Sotnikova et.al. "Effects of sesame oil in the model of adjuvant arthritis" *Neuro Endocrinol Lett.* 2009:30 Suppl 1:22-4 https://pubmed.ncbi.nlm.nih.gov/20027138/.

35 Deniz Senyilmaz-Tiebe et al. "Dietary stearic acid regulates mitochondria in vivo in humans. Nat Commun 9, 3129 (2018). https://doi.org/10.1038/s41467-018-05614-6.

36 Chris Woollams. "Conjugated linoleic acid, CLA, and cancer." https://www.canceractive.com/article/conjugated-linoleic-acid-cla-and-cancer.

37 Lisa Mulcahey."4 Research-Backed Health Benefits of Ghee." *Good Housekeeping.* https://www.goodhousekeeping.com/health/diet-nutrition/a64447254/health-benefits-of-ghee/.

Chapter 5: The Good Fats and Oils Shopping Guide and Resources

1 Diane Nelson. "Study Finds 82 Percent of Avocado Oil Rancid or Mixed With Other Oils." University of California, Davis. https://www.ucdavis.edu/food/news/study-finds-82-percent-avocado-oil-rancid-or-mixed-other-oils#:~:text=Wang%20and%20Hilary%20Green,%20a%20Ph.D.%20candidate.

2 "Olive Oil Brands To Avoid." FoodsGuy.com. https://foodsguy.com/olive-oil-brands-to-avoid/#:~:text=Olive%20oilis%20one%20of%20t.

3 "Pumpkin Seed Oil: Is It Good for You?" WebMD. https://www.webmd.com/diet/pumpkin-seed-oil-good-for-you.

4 Mira Miller. "What Happens to Your Body When You Take Pumpkin Seed Oil." verywellhealth (September 24, 2025). https://www.verywellhealth.com/pumpkin-seed-oil-benefits-11814378.

5 Lisa A. Kaminski. "What Is Cultured Butter and When Should You Use It?" *Taste of Home* (November 1, 2023). https://www.tasteofhome.com/article/what-is-cultured-butter/.

6 Annie Price. "Grass-Fed Butter: 7 Benefits That May Surprise You." Dr. Axe (October 28, 2024). https://draxe.com/nutrition/grass-fed-butter-nutrition/.

Index

#

4-HNE, 31
30-Minute Chicken Noodle Soup, recipe for, 86–87

A

acne, 40
Adventist Health Studies, 27
aggression, 44
almond oil
  benefits of individual oils and fats, 62
  healthy fats vs. unhealthy fats, 47
  shopping guide and resources for, 130
  smoke point of, 60, 61
alpha-linolenic acid (ALA), 38, 63. *See also* linoleic acid (LA)
Alzheimer's, 26, 31, 33, 38–40
American Heart Association, x, 8, 12, 51
animal fats. *See also* beef tallow; butter; ghee
  benefits of individual oils and fats, 64
  fatty acids in, 49
  healthy fats vs. unhealthy fats, 47
  shopping guide and resources for, 133–134
antidepressants, 33
Anti-Inflammatory Golden Milk, recipe for 119
antioxidants
  in black seed oil, 63
  in coconut oil, 62
  heart health and, 6
  in olive oil, 60
  seed oils and, 3, 15, 21, 22
anxiety, 34, 35–36
apolipoprotein A-IV (ApoA-IV), 61
appetite dysregulation, 43
arachidonic acid, 29, 40, 42
Avocado Chocolate Chip Cookies, recipe for, 102–103
avocado oil
  benefits of individual oils and fats, 62
  healthy fats vs. unhealthy fats, 47
  inflammation and, 45
  recipes with avocado oil, 99–104
  shopping guide and resources for, 129, 130
  smoke point of, 60, 61

B

beef tallow
  benefits of individual oils and fats, 64
  healthy fats vs. unhealthy fats, 47
  recipes with beef tallow, 127–128
  shopping guide and resources for, 129, 133
  smoke point of, 61
  use of, ix
Beet Brownies, recipe for, 101–102
benefits of individual oils and fats, 61–64
Big Fat Surprise, The (Teicholz), 10, 12
biofilms, 41
Black Bean, Corn, and Quinoa Salad, recipe for, 100–101
black cumin seed oil
  benefits of individual oils and fats, 63

healthy fats vs. unhealthy fats, 47
inflammation and, 45
toxic seed oils vs. healthy seed oils, 4
bleaching, 21
"blends" and vague terms, 18
brain health
blood-brain barrier, 31–32, 34
disrupted dopamine signals and, 33
disrupted neurotransmitter balance, 30
endocannabinoid system disruption, 31
fats and, 25–27, 45, 46–47
lipid peroxidation and brain cell damage, 31
microglial activation, 31
mitochondrial dysfunction, 31
neuroinflammation, 29–30
omega-6 and omega-3 imbalance and, 32–33
oxidative stress and toxic by-products and, 27–29
Bulletproof Coffee, recipe for, 110
butter
benefits of individual oils and fats, 64
healthy fats vs. unhealthy fats, 47
recipes with grass-fed butter, 110–118
shopping guide and resources for, 129, 133
smoke point of, 60, 61
Buttery Popcorn, recipe for, 111

C

Caesar Salad Dressing, recipe for, 68
Calbom, Cherie, 9, 11–12
calcium stearoyl, 57
cancer
benefits of individual oils and fats, 61, 62, 63
impact of diet on, 27
metabolic disruptions and, 43
omega-6 and omega-3 imbalance and, 32
oxidative stress and, 14, 15
seed oils and, x, 3, 25, 36–38
canola oil
creation of, 22–24
healthy fats vs. unhealthy fats, 48
homicide and aggression and, 44
seed oils, 3, 4, 13, 20, 56
where to find, 17
caprylic (C8) and capric (C10) acids, 63, 94
cardiovascular disease, 9, 10, 12, 15, 27, 43
Cauliflower Popcorn, recipe for, 72
Charlene's Cauliflower "Mashed Potatoes" with Spring Onions, recipe for, 125–126
Cheesy Dressing, recipe for, 68
chemical extraction, 22
Cherie's Best-Ever Garlic Butter Mashed Potatoes, recipe for, 114–115
Cherie's Ginger Lime Dressing, recipe for, 76
Cherie's Lemon Chicken Stir-Fry with Asparagus and Cherry Tomatoes, recipe for, 111–112
Cherie's Mint Marinade, recipe for, 77
Cherie's Old-Fashioned Beef Tallow Cornbread, recipe for, 127–128
Cherie's Simple Olive Oil Mayonnaise, recipe for, 76–77
Cheryl Hines's Whitefish with Lemon Caper Sauce, recipe for, 79–80
chia seed oil, 4, 32
Chocolate Superfood Balls, recipe for, 97–98
cholesterol
as "high cholesterol," 53–54
benefits of individual oils and fats, 62
cholesterol myth exposed, 52
dietary and blood cholesterol, 50

heart health and, 8, 9, 10, 28–29
inflammation and, 42
lipid hypothesis and, 55
myth vs. reality, 54
PUFAs and, 51
what we were taught, 5
cholesterol-free oil, 19
chronic inflammatory diseases, 32
Citrus Salad Dressing, recipe for, 68
Coconut Diet: The Secret Ingredient That Helps You Lose Weight While You Eat Your Favorite Foods, The (Calbom), 9
Coconut Lime Custard, recipe for, 90–91
coconut oil
benefits of individual oils and fats, 62
brain health and, 26
demonization of tropical oils, 49–50
healthy fats vs. unhealthy fats, 47
history, the lipid hypothesis, and the war on tropical oils, 54–56
recipes with coconut oil, 84–93
shopping guide and resources for, 131
smoke point of, 60, 61
cognitive decline, omega-3 deficiency, and Alzheimer's and dementia, 38–40
cold-pressed oils, 58
Comforting Creamy Tomato Soup, recipe for, 96–97
cooking oils at home, 17, 18
corn oil
healthy fats vs. unhealthy fats, 48
homicide and aggression and, 44
omega-6 and omega-3 imbalance and, 32, 33
seed oils, 3, 4, 13, 20
where to find, 17
cottonseed oil
healthy fats vs. unhealthy fats, 48
seed oils, 3, 4, 13, 19–20, 56
Country-Style Butter Piecrust, recipe for, 112–113
C-reactive proteins (CRP), 52
Cream of Carrot Soup, recipe for, 78
Creamy Avocado Dressing, recipe for, 68
Crisco, 1, 2, 12, 20

D

DATEM (diacetyl tartaric acid ester of mono- and diglycerides), 57
degumming, 21
dementia, x, 15, 26, 27, 31, 38–39
deodorization, 21–22
depression, 33, 34
DHA (docosahexaenoic acid), 26, 29, 30, 35, 38, 39, 132
diabetes, x, 5, 10, 20–21, 32, 33, 42, 43
dietary fats, four types of, 48–49
disrupted neurotransmitter balance, 30
DNA, x, 14, 15, 31, 34, 36, 37
dopamine, 33, 34
Dr. Jess's Golden Anti-Inflammatory Rice Bowls with Herby Lemon Chicken, recipe for, 122–124
Dr. Lake's Pumpkin Pancakes, recipe for, 120
Dr. Will Cole's Skillet Eggs with Spinach, recipe for, 121
dyslipidemia, 43

E

eczema, 40
egg lecithin, 57
emulsifiers, 19
endocannabinoid system disruption, 31, 34
EPA, 26, 29, 38
EPIC (European Prospective Investigation into Cancer and Nutrition), 27
erythrocyte sedimentation rate (ESR), 52
expeller-pressed oils, 58
extraction methods
cold-pressed, expeller-pressed, and solvent-extracted oils, 58
industrial processing of seed oils, 21–22

F

fats
- big fat lies, 11
- brain health and, 25–27
- dietary fats, four types of, 48–49
- essential fats, 58–59
- fat-soluble vitamins: why fat is a delivery system, 58
- healthy fats, 134
- heart-healthy myth and, 5–10
- individual fat tolerance, 64

fatty acids, 49. *See also specific types of*
fatty liver disease, 43
Feather-Light Coconut Macaroons, recipe for, 88–89
fish oil, 32, 49
Five-Spice Salmon, recipe for, 92–93
flaxseed oil
- benefits of individual oils and fats, 63
- brain health and, 25
- healthy fats vs. unhealthy fats, 47
- inflammation and, 45
- omega-6 and omega-3 imbalance and, 32
- practical guidelines for, 58
- shopping guide and resources for, 131
- toxic seed oils vs. healthy seed oils, 4
- what are seed oils, 3

Food Babe's No Sugar Granola by Vani Hari, recipe for, 91–92
fractionated oil, 57
frying oil, 18

G

Garlic Salad Dressing, recipe for, 68
George Foreman's Rosemary-Thyme Marinade, recipe for, 79
ghee
- benefits of individual oils and fats, 64
- healthy fats vs. unhealthy fats, 47
- recipes with ghee, 119–126
- shopping guide and resources for, 134
- smoke point of, 61

Ginger Salad Dressing, recipe for, 68
glucose dysregulation, 41–42, 43
Gluten-Free Shortbread Cookies, recipe for, 113–114
glycerin / glycerol esters of fatty acids, 57
Golden Rice, recipe for, 123
grapeseed oil
- healthy fats vs. unhealthy fats, 48
- seed oils, 3, 4, 56
- where to find, 17

Grass-Fed Beef Burritos/Tacos, recipe for, 70–72
Green Sprout Salad, recipe for, 73
Guacamole Greens Chicken Salad, recipe for, 73–75
gut barrier breakdown, 43

H

"hateful eight" oils, ix, 3, 56
Healing Strong's Mock Tuna Salad, recipe for, 103–104
healthy fats vs. unhealthy fats, 47–48
heart-healthy myth
- about seed oil scandal, 4–5
- foundations of heart health, 6–10
- what we now know, 6
- what we were taught, 5–6

heart-healthy oil, 19
"health-washed" names, 19
hemp seed oil
- benefits of individual oils and fats, 63
- healthy fats vs. unhealthy fats, 47
- shopping guide and resources for, 131
- toxic seed oils vs. healthy seed oils, 4
- what are seed oils, 3

hexane, 14, 20, 22, 52, 56, 58
history, the lipid hypothesis, and the war on tropical oils, 54–56
homicide and aggression, 44
Honey Mustard Dressing, recipe for, 68
hormone disruption and appetite dysregulation, 43

Hummus Salad Dressing, recipe for, 68
hydrogenated oil
  cleverly disguised names for seed oil, 57
  cottonseed oil and, 20
  omega-3 deficiencies and, 35
  processed-fat derivatives and, 18
  trans fats and, 49, 59
  use of, 55

I

immune disruption, 14
individual fat tolerance, 64
industrial processing of seed oils, 21–22
inflammation, 14, 15, 29–30, 34, 36, 42, 45
ingredients that often signal seed oils are present, 18–19
insulin resistance
  glucose dysregulation and, 41–42
  metabolic disruptions and, 43
  seed oils and, 15, 26, 33
  tumor development and, 37
  what we now know, 6
interesterified fats/oils, 18, 57

K

Kennedy, Robert F., Jr., 11, 24, 28
Keto-Friendly, Immunity-Boosting Fat Flush Soup, recipe for, 106–108
Kritchevsky, David, 12

L

LDL cholesterol, 28, 51, 62. *See also* cholesterol
lecithin, 18, 57
Lemon Garlic Marinade, recipe for, 112
Lemon-Herb Chicken, recipe for, 122
Liana's Basic Salad Dressing or Vinaigrette, recipe for, 67–68
Liana's OG 3-Hour Chicken Bone Broth Noodle Soup, recipe for, 94–95
life expectancy, reduction of, 32
light oil, 19
Lime Vinaigrette, recipe for, 68
linoleic acid (LA)
  brain health and, 26, 38
  cancer and, 32, 37
  depression and, 34, 36
  endocannabinoid system disruption and, 31
  homicide and aggression and, 44
  hormone disruption and, 43
  inflammation and, 29, 40, 42
  seed oils and, 14, 56
lipids
  lipid hypothesis, 8, 9, 50, 54–56
  lipid oxidation, storage, and rancidity, 58
  lipid peroxidation and brain cell damage, 31, 34
  lipid theory trap, 11–13
lipoproteins, 52, 53
long-chain fatty acids, 49, 56
Lundell, Dwight, 28–29, 33

M

macadamia nut oil
  benefits of individual oils and fats, 62
  healthy fats vs. unhealthy fats, 47
  recipes with macadamia nut oil, 105–108
  shopping guide and resources for, 131
  smoke point of, 60, 61
Macadamia Nut Salad, recipe for, 105–106
Mango Salad Dressing, recipe for, 68
margarine, 8, 13, 18, 35, 48, 51, 55, 59
Marla Maples's Gluten-Free Coconut Sugar Pecan Pie, recipe for, 116–117
MCT oil
  benefits of individual oils and fats, 63
  brain health and, 26
  recipes with MCT oil, 94–98
  shopping guide and resources for, 131–132
Mediterranean diet, 27, 39
medium-chain fatty acids, 49

metabolic issues, 41–42, 43–44
microglial activation, 31, 34
Mini Cashew Cheesecakes, recipe for, 87–88
Minnesota Coronary Experiment, 28
mitochondrial dysfunction, 31, 34, 43
modified vegetable oil, 57
Momma Mandy's White Bean Chicken Chili, recipe for, 115–116
mono- and diglycerides, 19, 57
monounsaturated fats, 26, 47, 48, 61, 62
mTORC1, 37
Mustard Vinaigrette, recipe for, 68

N

neurodegenerative conditions, 15, 27, 31, 38, 39
neuroinflammation, 29–30, 36
neurotransmitters, 34
neutralization, 21

O

obesity
- disrupted dopamine signals and, 33
- metabolic disruptions, 43
- omega-6 and omega-3 imbalance and, 33
- PUFAs and, 32
- seed oils and, x, 11, 15, 20
- weight gain, "sick fat," and obesity, 42
- what we were taught, 5

oleic sunflower oil/high oleic oil, 57
olive oil
- benefits of individual oils and fats, 61–62
- brain health and, 25, 26, 39–40
- healthy fats vs. unhealthy fats, 47
- inflammation and, 45
- recipes with olive oil, 67–83
- shopping guide and resources for, 129, 132
- smoke point of, 60, 61

omega-3 fatty acids
- anxiety and, 7, 34, 35–36
- in beef tallow, 133
- brain health and, 25, 26, 29, 38–40
- essential fats and, 58, 59
- in flaxseed oil, 63, 131
- in hempseed oil, 63, 131
- inflammation and, 40, 42, 47
- omega-6 and, 3, 14, 30, 31, 32–33, 50
- shopping guide and resources for, 132
- in walnut oil, 63, 133

omega-6 fatty acids
- anxiety and depression and, 34
- brain health and, 26, 30, 31, 33, 38
- colon cancer and, 37
- essential fats and, 58
- "health-washed" names, 19
- homicide and aggression and, 44
- inflammation and, 29, 30, 31, 34, 40, 41, 42
- omega-6 and omega-3 imbalance and, 32–33
- PUFAs and, 50
- seed oils and, 3, 14

oxidative stress and toxic by-products, 27–29

P

Paleo Hummingbird Muffins, recipe for, 117–118
palm oil, 56–57
palmitic acids (C16), 56
parasites, 41
Parkinson's, 31
peanut oil, 4, 48, 56
plant-based oil blends, 18
Plant-Based Taco Salad, recipe for, 69–70
polysorbates (e.g., polysorbate 80), 57
polyunsaturated fats (PUFAs)
- brain health and, 27–28, 29, 31, 51
- cancer and, 37
- dietary fats, four types of, 48–49
- heart health and, 28–29, 38
- lipid peroxidation and, 31
- omega-6 and omega-3 imbalance and, 32–33
- real cost of seed oils, 34

red flags of seed oil, 14
reverence of, 51–52
smoke point of, 60
truth about PUFAs revealed, 50–51
weight gain and, 43
processed-fat derivatives, 18
Proctor & Gamble, 12, 20
proprietary oil blends, 18
propylene glycol esters of fatty acids, 57
psoriasis, 40
pumpkin seed oil
benefits of individual oils and fats, 63
healthy fats vs. unhealthy fats, 47
shopping guide and resources for, 132
toxic seed oils vs. healthy seed oils, 4
what are seed oils, 3
Pumpkin Spice Oatmeal Balls, recipe for, 89–90
pure vegetable oil, 19

R

R. J. Reynolds Tobacco Company, 10
rapeseed
canola oil, creation of, 22–24
healthy fats vs. unhealthy fats, 48
seed oils, 2–3, 4, 57
real cost of seed oils, 34
Real Food Baked Pasta with Tomato, Herbs, and Mozzarella, recipe for, 82–83
recipe with sesame seed oil
Thai Chicken Super Salad, 109
ways to use sesame seed oil, 109
recipes with avocado oil
Avocado Chocolate Chip Cookies, 102–103
Beet Brownies, 101–102
Black Bean, Corn, and Quinoa Salad, 100–101
Healing Strong's Mock Tuna Salad, 103–104
Walnut-Crusted Chicken Tenders, 99–100
ways to use avocado oil, 99
recipes with beef tallow
Cherie's Old-Fashioned Beef Tallow Cornbread, 127–128
ways to use beef tallow, 127
recipes with coconut oil
30-Minute Chicken Noodle Soup, 86–87
Coconut Lime Custard, 90–91
Feather-Light Coconut Macaroons, 88–89
Five-Spice Salmon, 92–93
Food Babe's No Sugar Granola by Vani Hari, 91–92
Mini Cashew Cheesecakes, 87–88
Pumpkin Spice Oatmeal Balls, 89–90
Super-Speedy Supper, 85–86
Watercress Weight Loss Soup, 84–85
ways to use coconut oil, 84
recipes with ghee
Anti-Inflammatory Golden Milk, 119
Charlene's Cauliflower "Mashed Potatoes" with Spring Onions, 125–126
Dr. Jess's Golden Anti-Inflammatory Rice Bowls with Herby Lemon Chicken, 122–124
Dr. Lake's Pumpkin Pancakes, 120
Dr. Will Cole's Skillet Eggs with Spinach, 121
ways to use ghee, 119
recipes with grass-fed butter
Bulletproof Coffee, 110
Buttery Popcorn, 111
Cherie's Best-Ever Garlic Butter Mashed Potatoes, 114–115
Cherie's Lemon Chicken Stir-Fry with Asparagus and Cherry Tomatoes, 111–112
Country-Style Butter Piecrust, 112–113

- Gluten-Free Shortbread Cookies, 113–114
- Marla Maples's Gluten-Free Coconut Sugar Pecan Pie, 116–117
- Momma Mandy's White Bean Chicken Chili, 115–116
- Paleo Hummingbird Muffins, 117–118
- ways to use butter, 110

recipes with macadamia nut oil
- Keto-Friendly, Immunity-Boosting Fat Flush Soup, 106–108
- Macadamia Nut Salad, 105–106
- ways to use macadamia nut oil, 105

recipes with MCT oil
- Chocolate Superfood Balls, 97–98
- Comforting Creamy Tomato Soup, 96–97
- Liana's OG 3-Hour Chicken Bone Broth Noodle Soup, 94–95
- ways to use MCT oil, 94

recipes with nature's healthiest fats and oils
- about, 65
- tips for healthy cooking, 66

recipes with olive oil
- Cauliflower Popcorn, 72
- Cherie's Ginger Lime Dressing, 76
- Cherie's Mint Marinade, 77
- Cherie's Simple Olive Oil Mayonnaise, 76–77
- Cheryl Hines's Whitefish with Lemon Caper Sauce, 79–80
- Cream of Carrot Soup, 78
- George Foreman's Rosemary-Thyme Marinade, 79
- Grass-Fed Beef Burritos/Tacos, 70–72
- Green Sprout Salad, 73
- Guacamole Greens Chicken Salad, 73–75
- Liana's Basic Salad Dressing or Vinaigrette, 67–68
- Plant-Based Taco Salad, 69–70
- Real Food Baked Pasta with Tomato, Herbs, and Mozzarella, 82–83
- Sourdough Bread Pizza with Grass-Fed Beef and Buffalo Mozzarella, 81
- Superfood Kale Salad, 75
- ways to use olive oil, 67

restaurant cooking
- red flags of seed oil, 14
- resources for shopping and eating out, 134–136
- where to find seed oils, 16

rice bran oil, 4, 17, 48, 56

Roasted Sunflower Seed Dressing, recipe for, 68

S

safflower oil
- cancer and, 37
- healthy fats vs. unhealthy fats, 48
- what are seed oils, 3, 4, 20, 56
- where to find, 17

saturated fats
- heart health and, 4, 8, 9, 28–29, 50
- lipid hypothesis and, 55
- lipid theory and, 12
- PUFAs and, 51
- saturated and unsaturated fats, setting the record straight, 49
- types of dietary fats, 48

seed oil industry
- canola oil, creation of, 22–24
- industrial processing of seed oils, 21–22
- projected earnings of, xi
- spiritual aspects of food and, xi

seed oils
- about, 2–3
- "blends" and vague terms, 18

change and, 24
cleverly disguised names for, 57
dark history of, 19–21
heart-healthy myth, 4–11
"health-washed" names, 19
industrial processing of, 21–22
ingredients that often signal, 18–19
lipid theory trap, 11–13
oils not recommended for use, 56–57
prevalence and assumptions about, x
processed-fat derivatives, 18
real cost of seed oils, 34
red flags of seed oil, 13–15
seed oil scandal, 1–24
toxic seed oils vs. healthy seed oils, 4
where to find, 16–18

Sesame Ginger Dressing, recipe for, 69

sesame seed oil
benefits of individual oils and fats, 63
recipe with sesame seed oil, 109
shopping guide and resources for, 133
smoke point of, 61
toxic seed oils vs. healthy seed oils, 4
what are seed oils, 3

Shanahan, C., 53

shopping guide and resources for
animal fats, 133–134
oils for your kitchen, 130–133
resources for shopping and eating out, 134–136
tips in a nutshell, 129–130
virgin and extra-virgin oil, 130

short-chain fatty acids (SCFAs), 38

shortening, 18, 20, 35, 48, 55, 59

"sick fat," 42

skin, impact of seed oil on, 40

smoke points of fats and oils, 60–61

smoking, 8, 10, 50, 52, 55, 60

solvent-extracted oils, 58

sorbitan monostearate, 57

Sourdough Bread Pizza with Grass-Fed Beef and Buffalo Mozzarella, recipe for, 81

soy lecithin, 18, 57

soybean oil
healthy fats vs. unhealthy fats, 48
homicide and aggression and, 44
omega-6 and omega-3 imbalance and, 32
seed oils, 2, 4, 13, 20, 56
where to find, 17

Spicy Salad Dressing, recipe for, 69

spiritual aspects of food, xi

SSL (sodium stearoyl-2-lactylate), 57

stearates, 57

stearic acids (C18), 56, 64

Stein, John, 33

storing oils, guidelines for, 58

sucrose esters, 57

sunflower oil
healthy fats vs. unhealthy fats, 48
omega-6 and omega-3 imbalance and, 33
seed oils, 4, 20, 56, 57
where to find, 17

Superfood Kale Salad, recipe for, 75

Super-Speedy Supper, recipe for, 85–86

Sweet Salad Dressing, recipe for, 69

T

Tahini Salad Dressing, recipe for, 69

Teicholz, Nina, 10, 12

Thai Curry Dressing, recipe for, 69

tigernut oil, 47

tocopherols (vitamin E), 57

toxic seed oils vs. healthy seed oils, 4

trans fats
as dangerous industrial creation, 59
dietary fats, four types of, 49
healthy fats vs. unhealthy fats, 48
impact of, 35–36, 47

tropical oils. *See also* coconut oil
- demonization of, 49–50
- history, the lipid hypothesis, and the war on tropical oils, 54–56

Turmeric Salad Dressing, recipe for, 69
twelve red flags of seed oil, 13–15

U

unsaturated fats, 39, 49, 51, 59

V

vegetable oils. *See also* seed oils
- "blends" and vague terms, 18
- cleverly disguised names for seed oil, 57
- healthy fats vs. unhealthy fats, 48
- use of term, x, 2
- where to find, 17

vitamins, fat-soluble vitamins, 58

W

Walnut-Crusted Chicken Tenders, recipe for, 99–100
walnut oil
- benefits of individual oils and fats, 63
- healthy fats vs. unhealthy fats, 47
- shopping guide and resources for, 133

Watercress Weight Loss Soup, recipe for, 84–85